About us

Name: _____

Name: _____

Age: _____

Age: _____

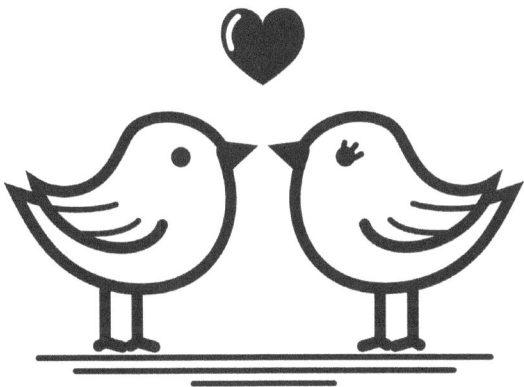

Together since

_____ / ____ / _____

How we met

_____

_____

_____

_____

Table of contents

Important facts:

How do you figure out when you're fertile and when you're not?

Being aware of your menstrual cycle and the changes in your body that happen during this time can help you know when you are most likely to get pregnant.

The average menstrual cycle lasts 28 days. But normal cycles can vary from 21 to 35 days. The amount of time before ovulation occurs is different in every woman and even can be different from month to month in the same woman, varying from 13 to 20 days long. Learning about this part of the cycle is important because it is when ovulation and pregnancy can occur. After ovulation, every woman (unless she has a health problem that affects her periods or becomes pregnant) will have a period within 14 to 16 days.

Knowing when you're most fertile will help you plan pregnancy. There are three ways you can keep track of your fertile times. They are:

- **Basal body temperature method** – Basal body temperature is your temperature at rest as soon as you awake in the morning. A woman's basal body temperature rises slightly with ovulation. So by recording this temperature daily for several months, you'll be able to predict your most fertile days.

Basal body temperature differs slightly from woman to woman. Anywhere from 96 to 98 degrees Fahrenheit orally is average before ovulation. After ovulation most women have an oral temperature between 97 and 99 degrees Fahrenheit. The rise in temperature can be a sudden jump or a gradual climb over a few days.

Usually a woman's basal body temperature rises by only 0.4 to 0.8 degrees Fahrenheit. To detect this tiny change, women must use a basal body thermometer. These thermometers are very sensitive. Most pharmacies sell them for about $10.

The rise in temperature doesn't show exactly when the egg is released. But almost all women have ovulated within three days after their temperatures spike. Body temperature stays at the higher level until your period starts.

You are most fertile and most likely to get pregnant:

- Two to three days before your temperature hits the highest point (ovulation)
- and
- 12 to 24 hours after ovulation

A man's sperm can live for up to three days in a woman's body. The sperm can fertilize an egg at any point during that time. So if you have unprotected sex a few days before ovulation, you could get pregnant.

Many things can affect basal body temperature. For your chart to be useful, make sure to take your temperature every morning at about the same time. Things that can alter your temperature include:

- Drinking alcohol the night before
- Smoking cigarettes the night before
- Getting a poor night's sleep
- Having a fever
- Doing anything in the morning before you take your temperature — including going to the bathroom and talking on the phone

- **Calendar method** – This involves recording your menstrual cycle on a calendar for eight to 12 months. The first day of your period is Day 1. Circle Day 1 on the calendar. The length of your cycle may vary from month to month. So write down the total number of days it lasts each time. Using this record, you can find the days you are most fertile in the months ahead:

1.To find out the first day when you are most fertile, subtract 18 from the total number of days in your shortest cycle. Take this new number and count ahead that many days from the first day of your next period. Draw an X through this date on your calendar. The X marks the first day you're likely to be fertile.

2.To find out the last day when you are most fertile, subtract 11 from the total number of days in your longest cycle. Take this new number and count ahead that many days from the first day of your next period. Draw an X through this date on your calendar. The time between the two Xs is your most fertile window.

This method always should be used along with other fertility awareness methods, especially if your cycles are not always the same length.

- **Cervical mucus method (also known as the ovulation method)** – This involves being aware of the changes in your cervical mucus throughout the month. The hormones that control the menstrual cycle also change the kind and amount of mucus you have before and during ovulation. Right after your period, there are usually a few days when there is no mucus present or "dry days." As the egg starts to mature, mucus increases in the vagina, appears at the vaginal opening, and is white or yellow and cloudy and sticky. The greatest amount of mucus appears just before ovulation. During these "wet days" it becomes clear and slippery, like raw egg whites. Sometimes it can be stretched apart. This is when you are most fertile. About four days after the wet days begin the mucus changes again. There will be much less and it becomes sticky and cloudy. You might have a few more dry days before your period returns. Describe changes in your mucus on a calendar. Label the days, "Sticky," "Dry," or "Wet." You are most fertile at the first sign of wetness after your period or a day or two before wetness begins.

The cervical mucus method is less reliable for some women. Women who are breastfeeding, taking hormonal birth control (like the pill), using feminine hygiene products, have vaginitis or sexually transmitted infections (STIs), or have had surgery on the cervix should not rely on this method.

- To most accurately track your fertility, use a combination of all three methods. This is called the symptothermal method. You can also purchase over-the-counter ovulation kits or fertility monitors to help find the best time to conceive. These kits work by detecting surges in a specific hormone called luteinizing hormone, which triggers ovulation.

What are the signs of Ovulation?
- Rise in basal body temperature, typically 1/2 to 1 degree, measured by a thermometer
- Higher levels of luteinizing hormone (LH), measured on a home ovulation kit
- Cervical mucus, or vaginal discharge, may appear clearer, thinner, and stretchy, like raw egg whites
- Breast tenderness
- Bloating
- Light spotting
- Slight pain or cramping in your side

Tips for Conception

- ◯ take prenatals & folic acid

- ◯ reduce caffeine intake

- ◯ drink lots of water

- ◯ start self care routine

- ◯ stop recreational drugs & check prescriptions

- ◯ establish healthy eating habits

- ◯ avoid eating fish high in mercury

- ◯ maintain a healthy weight & bmi

- ◯ stop drinking alcohol

- ◯ track cycle & ovulation

- ◯ get a routine physical

- ◯ go to the dentist

- ◯ stop birth control

Cycle Tracker

	Jan	Feb	Mar	Apr	May	Jun	Jul	Aug	Sep	Oct	Nov	Dec
1	○	○	○	○	○	○	○	○	○	○	○	○
2	○	○	○	○	○	○	○	○	○	○	○	○
3	○	○	○	○	○	○	○	○	○	○	○	○
4	○	○	○	○	○	○	○	○	○	○	○	○
5	○	○	○	○	○	○	○	○	○	○	○	○
6	○	○	○	○	○	○	○	○	○	○	○	○
7	○	○	○	○	○	○	○	○	○	○	○	○
8	○	○	○	○	○	○	○	○	○	○	○	○
9	○	○	○	○	○	○	○	○	○	○	○	○
10	○	○	○	○	○	○	○	○	○	○	○	○
11	○	○	○	○	○	○	○	○	○	○	○	○
12	○	○	○	○	○	○	○	○	○	○	○	○
13	○	○	○	○	○	○	○	○	○	○	○	○
14	○	○	○	○	○	○	○	○	○	○	○	○
15	○	○	○	○	○	○	○	○	○	○	○	○
16	○	○	○	○	○	○	○	○	○	○	○	○
17	○	○	○	○	○	○	○	○	○	○	○	○
18	○	○	○	○	○	○	○	○	○	○	○	○
19	○	○	○	○	○	○	○	○	○	○	○	○
20	○	○	○	○	○	○	○	○	○	○	○	○
21	○	○	○	○	○	○	○	○	○	○	○	○
22	○	○	○	○	○	○	○	○	○	○	○	○
23	○	○	○	○	○	○	○	○	○	○	○	○
24	○	○	○	○	○	○	○	○	○	○	○	○
25	○	○	○	○	○	○	○	○	○	○	○	○
26	○	○	○	○	○	○	○	○	○	○	○	○
27	○	○	○	○	○	○	○	○	○	○	○	○
28	○	○	○	○	○	○	○	○	○	○	○	○
29	○	○	○	○	○	○	○	○	○	○	○	○
30	○	○	○	○	○	○	○	○	○	○	○	○
31	○	○	○	○	○	○	○	○	○	○	○	○

Cycle tracker

first day of period _____

cycle number _____

January

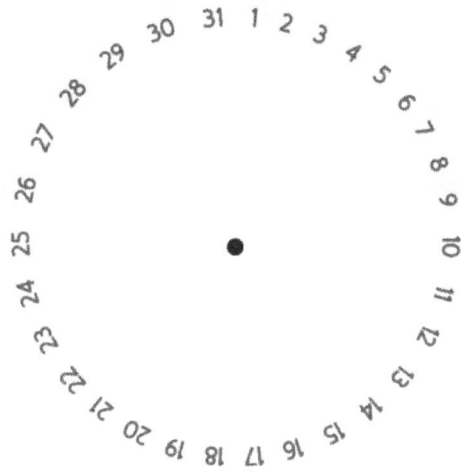

Menstruation Flow

Day 1	Day 2	Day 3
○○○○○	○○○○○	○○○○○

Day 4	Day 5	Day 6
○○○○○	○○○○○	○○○○○

Day 7

○○○○○

Mood

Day 1	Day 2	Day 3	Day 4	Day 5	Day 6	Day 7
calm	calm	calm	calm	calm	calm	calm
happy	happy	happy	happy	happy	happy	happy
energetic	energetic	energetic	energetic	energetic	energetic	energetic
irritated	irritated	irritated	irritated	irritated	irritated	irritated
sad	sad	sad	sad	sad	sad	sad
anxious	anxious	anxious	anxious	anxious	anxious	anxious

Symptoms

Day 1	Day 2	Day 3	Day 4	Day 5	Day 6	Day 7
acne	acne	acne	acne	acne	acne	acne
nausea	nausea	nausea	nausea	nausea	nausea	nausea
cramps	cramps	cramps	cramps	cramps	cramps	cramps
headache	headache	headache	headache	headache	headache	headache
fatigue	fatigue	fatigue	fatigue	fatigue	fatigue	fatigue
bloating	bloating	bloating	bloating	bloating	bloating	bloating
back ache	back ache	back ache	back ache	back ache	back ache	back ache
sore boobs	sore boobs	sore boobs	sore boobs	sore boobs	sore boobs	sore boobs

Sleep
_____

Weight
_____

Water
_____

1
2
3
4
5
6
7
8
9
10
11
12
13
14
15
16
17
18
19
20
21
22
23
24
25
26
27
28
29
30
31

Notes:

Date _____

Daily Cycle Log

Cycle Day _____

temperature _____ opk result _____ cervical fluid _____
(none, sticky, egg white, watery, unusual)

my mood today is...

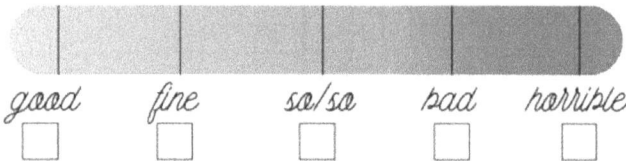

good   fine   so/so   bad   horrible
☐   ☐   ☐   ☐   ☐

thoughts about how i'm feeling :

_____

_____

_____

_____

water intake tracker

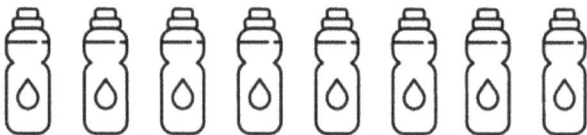

exercise

meals for the day

prenatal vitamin ☑

breakfast_____

lunch_____

dinner_____

snacks_____

Intercourse

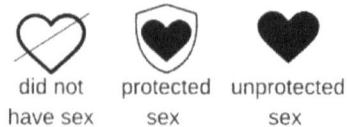

did not have sex   protected sex   unprotected sex

Mood

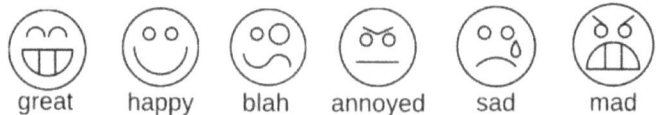

great   happy   blah   annoyed   sad   mad

Symptoms

tender breasts	headache	backache	fatigue	cravings
cramps	acne	nausea	bloating	insomnia
constipation	diarrhea	joint pain	spotting	congestion

Date _____ # Daily Cycle Log Cycle Day _____

temperature _____ opk result _____ cervical fluid _____
(none, sticky, egg white, watery, unusual)

my mood today is...

good *fine* *so/so* *bad* *horrible*
☐ ☐ ☐ ☐ ☐

water intake tracker

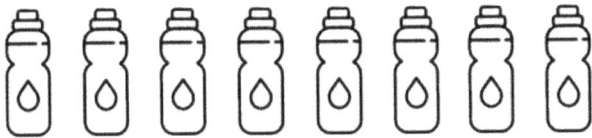

meals for the day

breakfast _____

lunch _____

dinner _____

snacks _____

thoughts about how i'm feeling :

_____

_____

_____

_____

exercise

prenatal vitamin ☑

Intercourse

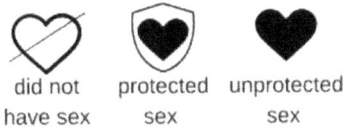

did not have sex   protected sex   unprotected sex

Mood

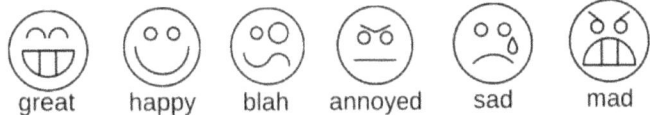

great   happy   blah   annoyed   sad   mad

Symptoms

tender breasts	headache	backache	fatigue	cravings
cramps	acne	nausea	bloating	insomnia
constipation	diarrhea	joint pain	spotting	congestion

Date _____ # Daily Cycle Log Cycle Day_____

temperature _____ opk result _____ cervical fluid _____
(none, sticky, egg white, watery, unusual)

my mood today is...

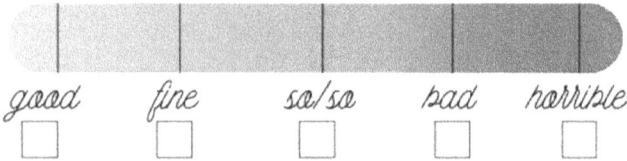

good   *fine*   *so/so*   *bad*   *horrible*
☐   ☐   ☐   ☐   ☐

thoughts about how i'm feeling :

_____
_____
_____
_____

water intake tracker

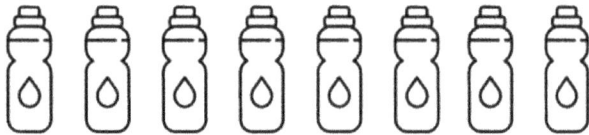

exercise

meals for the day   prenatal vitamin ☑

*breakfast*_____

*lunch*_____

*dinner*_____

*snacks*_____

Intercourse

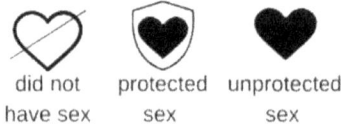

did not   protected   unprotected
have sex   sex   sex

Mood

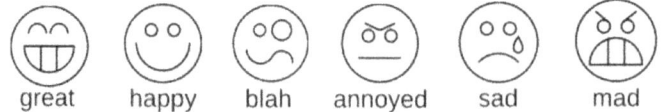

great   happy   blah   annoyed   sad   mad

Symptoms

tender breasts	headache	backache	fatigue	cravings
cramps	acne	nausea	bloating	insomnia
constipation	diarrhea	joint pain	spotting	congestion

Date _____   # Daily Cycle Log   Cycle Day _____

temperature _____   opk result _____   cervical fluid _____
(none, sticky, egg white, watery, unusual)

my mood today is...

good   fine   so/so   bad   horrible
☐   ☐   ☐   ☐   ☐

thoughts about how i'm feeling :

_____

_____

_____

_____

water intake tracker

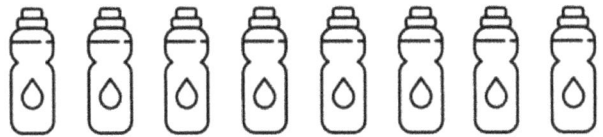

exercise

meals for the day

prenatal vitamin ☑

breakfast _____

lunch _____

dinner _____

snacks _____

Intercourse

did not have sex   protected sex   unprotected sex

Mood

great   happy   blah   annoyed   sad   mad

Symptoms

tender breasts	headache	backache	fatigue	cravings
cramps	acne	nausea	bloating	insomnia
constipation	diarrhea	joint pain	spotting	congestion

Daily Cycle Log

Date _____

Cycle Day_____

temperature _____   opk result_____   cervical fluid _____

(none, sticky, egg white, watery, unusual)

my mood today is...

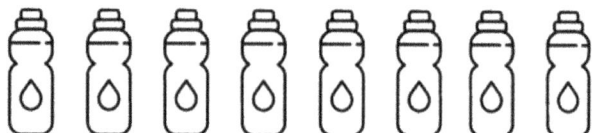

good   fine   so/so   bad   horrible
☐   ☐   ☐   ☐   ☐

thoughts about how i'm feeling :

_____

_____

_____

_____

water intake tracker

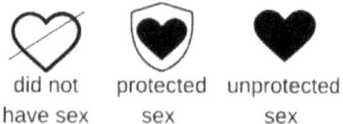

exercise

_____

meals for the day

prenatal vitamin ▢

breakfast_____

lunch_____

dinner_____

snacks_____

Intercourse

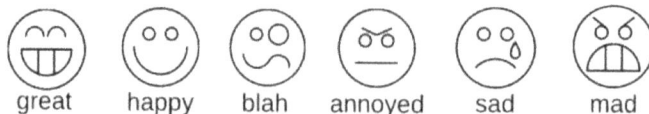

did not have sex   protected sex   unprotected sex

Mood

great   happy   blah   annoyed   sad   mad

Symptoms

tender breasts	headache	backache	fatigue	cravings
cramps	acne	nausea	bloating	insomnia
constipation	diarrhea	joint pain	spotting	congestion

Date _____   # Daily Cycle Log   Cycle Day_____

temperature _____   opk result _____   cervical fluid _____
(none, sticky, egg white, watery, unusual)

my mood today is...

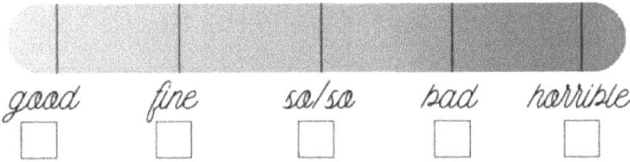

good   *fine*   *so/so*   *bad*   *horrible*
☐   ☐   ☐   ☐   ☐

water intake tracker

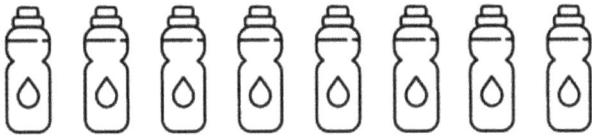

meals for the day

thoughts about how i'm feeling :

_____
_____
_____
_____

exercise

prenatal vitamin ▢

*breakfast*_____

*lunch*_____

*dinner*_____

*snacks*_____

Intercourse

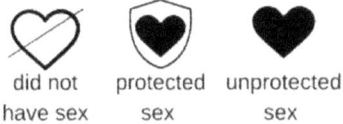

did not   protected   unprotected
have sex   sex   sex

Mood

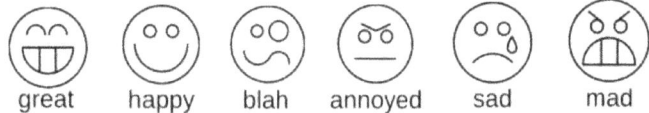

great   happy   blah   annoyed   sad   mad

Symptoms

tender breasts	headache	backache	fatigue	cravings
cramps	acne	nausea	bloating	insomnia
constipation	diarrhea	joint pain	spotting	congestion

Date _____ # Daily Cycle Log Cycle Day _____

temperature _____   opk result _____   cervical fluid _____
(none, sticky, egg white, watery, unusual)

my mood today is...

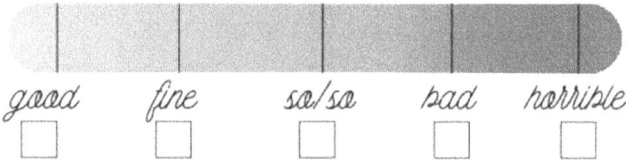

good   fine   so/so   bad   horrible
☐   ☐   ☐   ☐   ☐

water intake tracker

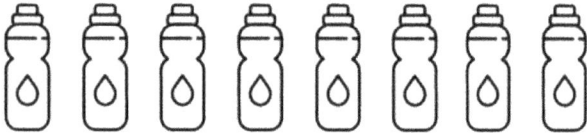

thoughts about how i'm feeling :

_____
_____
_____
_____

exercise
_____
| |
| |
| |
|_____|

prenatal vitamin 🔲

meals for the day

breakfast _____

lunch _____

dinner _____

snacks _____

Intercourse

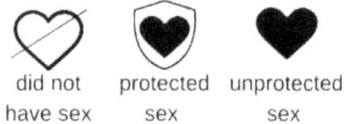

did not   protected   unprotected
have sex   sex   sex

Mood

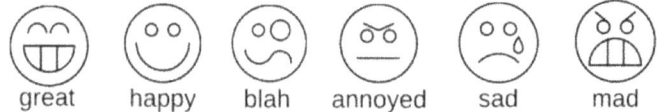

great   happy   blah   annoyed   sad   mad

Symptoms

tender breasts	headache	backache	fatigue	cravings
cramps	acne	nausea	bloating	insomnia
constipation	diarrhea	joint pain	spotting	congestion

basal body temperature chart

date range _____

cycle # _____

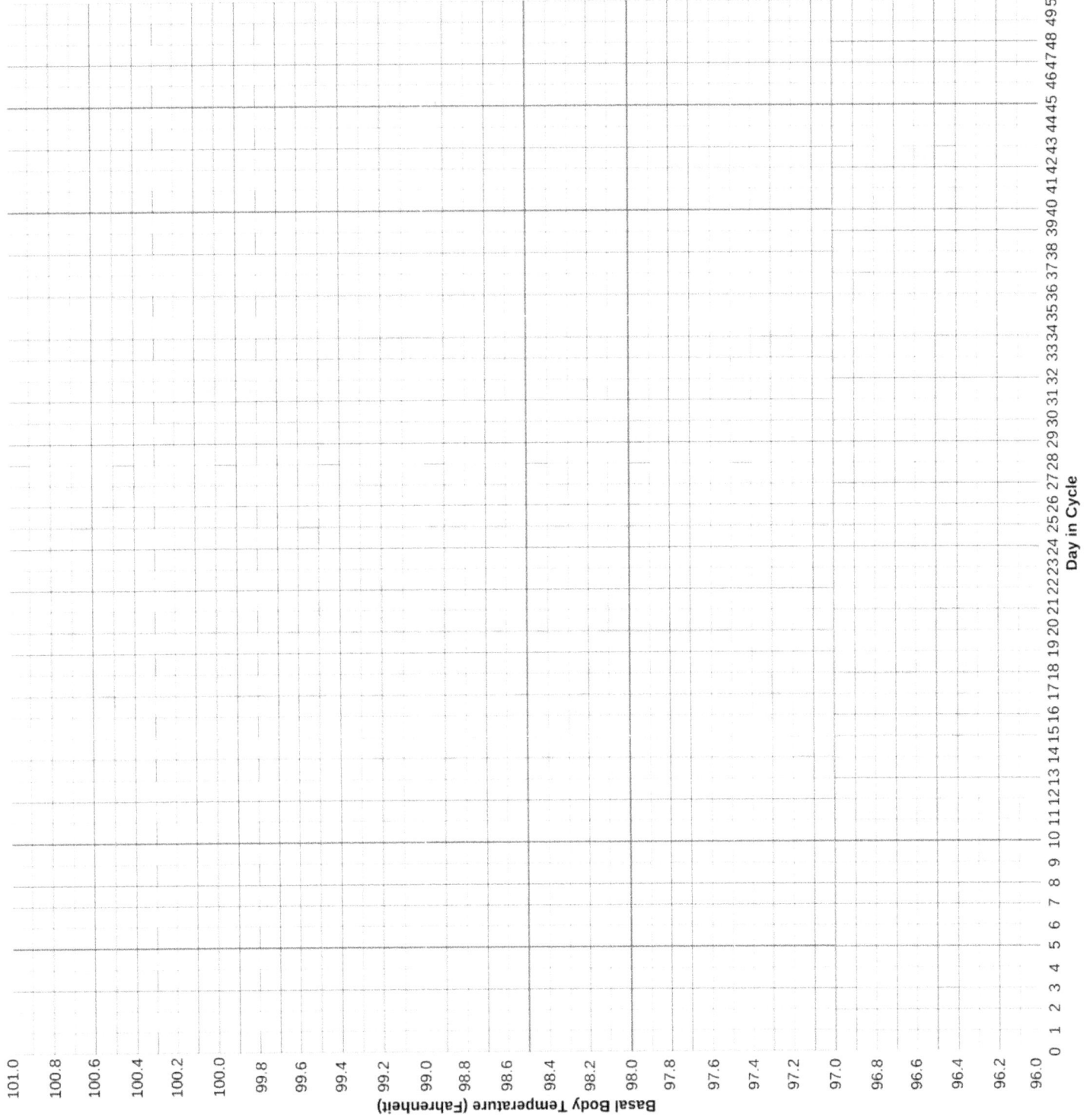

Basal Body Temperature (Fahrenheit)

101.0
100.8
100.6
100.4
100.2
100.0
99.8
99.6
99.4
99.2
99.0
98.8
98.6
98.4
98.2
98.0
97.8
97.6
97.4
97.2
97.0
96.8
96.6
96.4
96.2
96.0

0 1 2 3 4 5 6 7 8 9 10 11 12 13 14 15 16 17 18 19 20 21 22 23 24 25 26 27 28 29 30 31 32 33 34 35 36 37 38 39 40 41 42 43 44 45 46 47 48 49 50

Day in Cycle

Cycle tracker

first day of period _____

cycle number _____

February

Menstruation Flow

Day 1	Day 2	Day 3
○○○○○	○○○○○	○○○○○

Day 4	Day 5	Day 6
○○○○○	○○○○○	○○○○○

Day 7

○○○○○

Mood

Day 1	Day 2	Day 3	Day 4	Day 5	Day 6	Day 7
calm	calm	calm	calm	calm	calm	calm
happy	happy	happy	happy	happy	happy	happy
energetic	energetic	energetic	energetic	energetic	energetic	energetic
irritated	irritated	irritated	irritated	irritated	irritated	irritated
sad	sad	sad	sad	sad	sad	sad
anxious	anxious	anxious	anxious	anxious	anxious	anxious

Symptoms

Day 1	Day 2	Day 3	Day 4	Day 5	Day 6	Day 7
acne	acne	acne	acne	acne	acne	acne
nausea	nausea	nausea	nausea	nausea	nausea	nausea
cramps	cramps	cramps	cramps	cramps	cramps	cramps
headache	headache	headache	headache	headache	headache	headache
fatigue	fatigue	fatigue	fatigue	fatigue	fatigue	fatigue
bloating	bloating	bloating	bloating	bloating	bloating	bloating
back ache	back ache	back ache	back ache	back ache	back ache	back ache
sore boobs	sore boobs	sore boobs	sore boobs	sore boobs	sore boobs	sore boobs

Sleep

Weight

Water

1	
2	
3	
4	
5	
6	
7	
8	
9	
10	
11	
12	
13	
14	
15	
16	
17	
18	
19	
20	
21	
22	
23	
24	
25	
26	
27	
28	
29	
30	
31	

Notes:

Daily Cycle Log

Date _____   Cycle Day _____

temperature _____   opk result _____   cervical fluid _____
(none, sticky, egg white, watery, unusual)

my mood today is...

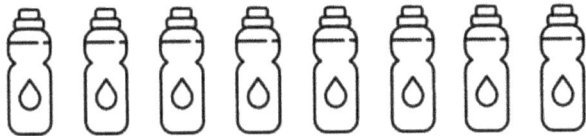

good   fine   so/so   bad   horrible
☐   ☐   ☐   ☐   ☐

water intake tracker

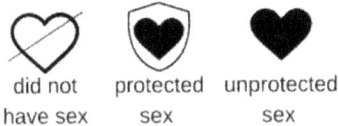

thoughts about how i'm feeling :

_____
_____
_____
_____

exercise

prenatal vitamin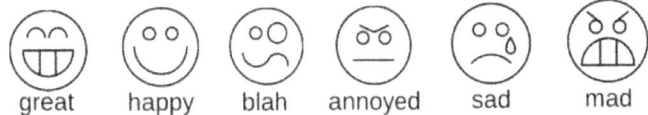

meals for the day

breakfast _____

lunch _____

dinner _____

snacks _____

Intercourse

did not have sex   protected sex   unprotected sex

Mood

great   happy   blah   annoyed   sad   mad

Symptoms

tender breasts	headache	backache	fatigue	cravings
cramps	acne	nausea	bloating	insomnia
constipation	diarrhea	joint pain	spotting	congestion

Daily Cycle Log

Date _____   Cycle Day_____

temperature _____   opk result _____   cervical fluid _____
(none, sticky, egg white, watery, unusual)

my mood today is...

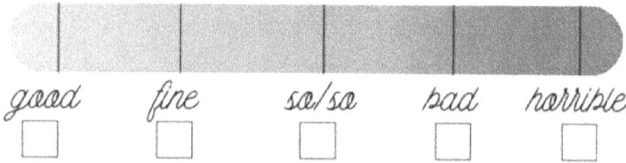

good   *fine*   *so/so*   *bad*   *horrible*
☐   ☐   ☐   ☐   ☐

thoughts about how i'm feeling :

_____
_____
_____
_____

water intake tracker

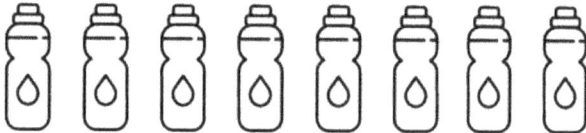

exercise

prenatal vitamin ☑

meals for the day

breakfast _____

lunch _____

dinner _____

snacks _____

Intercourse

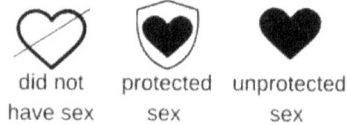

did not have sex   protected sex   unprotected sex

Mood

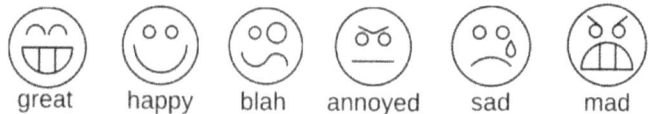

great   happy   blah   annoyed   sad   mad

Symptoms

tender breasts	headache	backache	fatigue	cravings
cramps	acne	nausea	bloating	insomnia
constipation	diarrhea	joint pain	spotting	congestion

Daily Cycle Log

Date _____   Cycle Day_____

temperature _____   opk result_____   cervical fluid _____
(none, sticky, egg white, watery, unusual)

my mood today is...

good ☐   fine ☐   so/so ☐   bad ☐   horrible ☐

thoughts about how i'm feeling :

_____
_____
_____
_____

water intake tracker

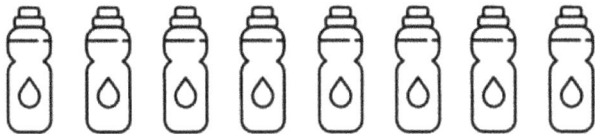

exercise

meals for the day

prenatal vitamin

breakfast _____

lunch _____

dinner _____

snacks _____

Intercourse

did not have sex   protected sex   unprotected sex

Mood

great   happy   blah   annoyed   sad   mad

Symptoms

tender breasts	headache	backache	fatigue	cravings
cramps	acne	nausea	bloating	insomnia
constipation	diarrhea	joint pain	spotting	congestion

Date _____ # Daily Cycle Log Cycle Day _____

temperature _____   opk result _____   cervical fluid _____
(none, sticky, egg white, watery, unusual)

my mood today is...

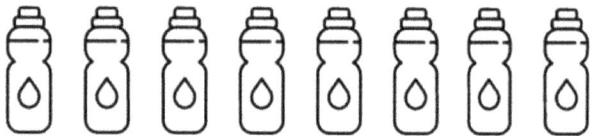

good   fine   so/so   bad   horrible
☐   ☐   ☐   ☐   ☐

thoughts about how i'm feeling :

_____

_____

_____

_____

water intake tracker

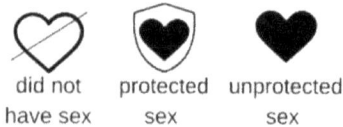

exercise

meals for the day

prenatal vitamin ☐

breakfast _____

lunch _____

dinner _____

snacks _____

Intercourse

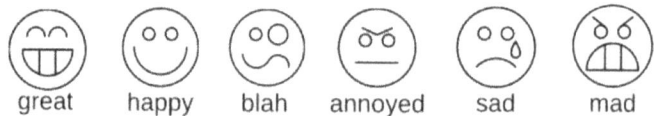

did not have sex   protected sex   unprotected sex

Mood

great   happy   blah   annoyed   sad   mad

Symptoms

tender breasts	headache	backache	fatigue	cravings
cramps	acne	nausea	bloating	insomnia
constipation	diarrhea	joint pain	spotting	congestion

Date _____ # Daily Cycle Log Cycle Day _____

temperature _____   opk result _____   cervical fluid _____
(none, sticky, egg white, watery, unusual)

my mood today is...

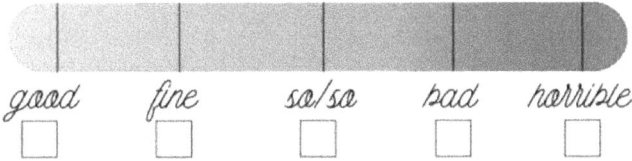

good   fine   so/so   bad   horrible
☐   ☐   ☐   ☐   ☐

water intake tracker

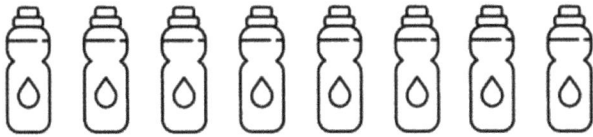

thoughts about how i'm feeling :

_____

_____

_____

_____

exercise

meals for the day

prenatal vitamin ☐

breakfast _____

lunch _____

dinner _____

snacks _____

Intercourse

did not   protected   unprotected
have sex   sex   sex

Mood

great   happy   blah   annoyed   sad   mad

Symptoms

tender breasts	headache	backache	fatigue	cravings
cramps	acne	nausea	bloating	insomnia
constipation	diarrhea	joint pain	spotting	congestion

Date _____   # Daily Cycle Log   Cycle Day _____

temperature _____   opk result _____   cervical fluid _____
                                                                (none, sticky, egg white, watery, unusual)

my mood today is...   thoughts about how i'm feeling :

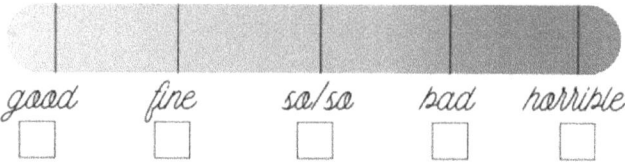

good   fine   so/so   bad   horrible
☐   ☐   ☐   ☐   ☐
                                             _____

                                             _____

water intake tracker   _____

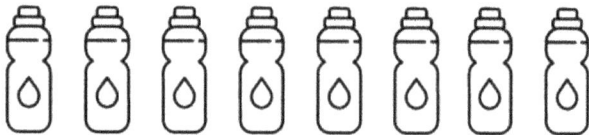

                                             _____

                                             ┌─────────────────────────────┐
                                             │ exercise   │
                                             │   │
                                             │   │
                                             │   │
                                             └─────────────────────────────┘

meals for the day   prenatal vitamin ▢

breakfast_____

lunch_____

dinner_____

snacks_____

Intercourse   ### Mood

did not   protected   unprotected   great   happy   blah   annoyed   sad   mad
have sex   sex   sex

Symptoms

tender breasts	headache	backache	fatigue	cravings
cramps	acne	nausea	bloating	insomnia
constipation	diarrhea	joint pain	spotting	congestion

Date _____ # Daily Cycle Log Cycle Day_____

temperature _____ opk result_____ cervical fluid _____
(none, sticky, egg white, watery, unusual)

my mood today is...

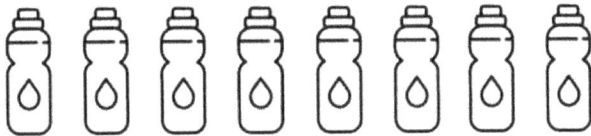

good   fine   so/so   bad   horrible
☐   ☐   ☐   ☐   ☐

water intake tracker

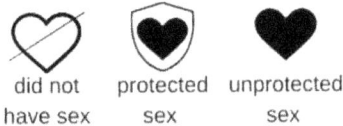

thoughts about how i'm feeling :

_____
_____
_____
_____

exercise

prenatal vitamin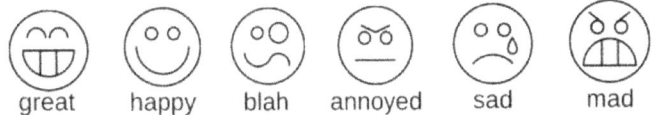

meals for the day

breakfast_____

lunch_____

dinner_____

snacks_____

Intercourse

did not have sex   protected sex   unprotected sex

Mood

great   happy   blah   annoyed   sad   mad

Symptoms

tender breasts	headache	backache	fatigue	cravings
cramps	acne	nausea	bloating	insomnia
constipation	diarrhea	joint pain	spotting	congestion

basal body Temperature chart

Basal Body Temperature (Fahrenheit)

101.0
100.8
100.6
100.4
100.2
100.0
99.8
99.6
99.4
99.2
99.0
98.8
98.6
98.4
98.2
98.0
97.8
97.6
97.4
97.2
97.0
96.8
96.6
96.4
96.2
96.0

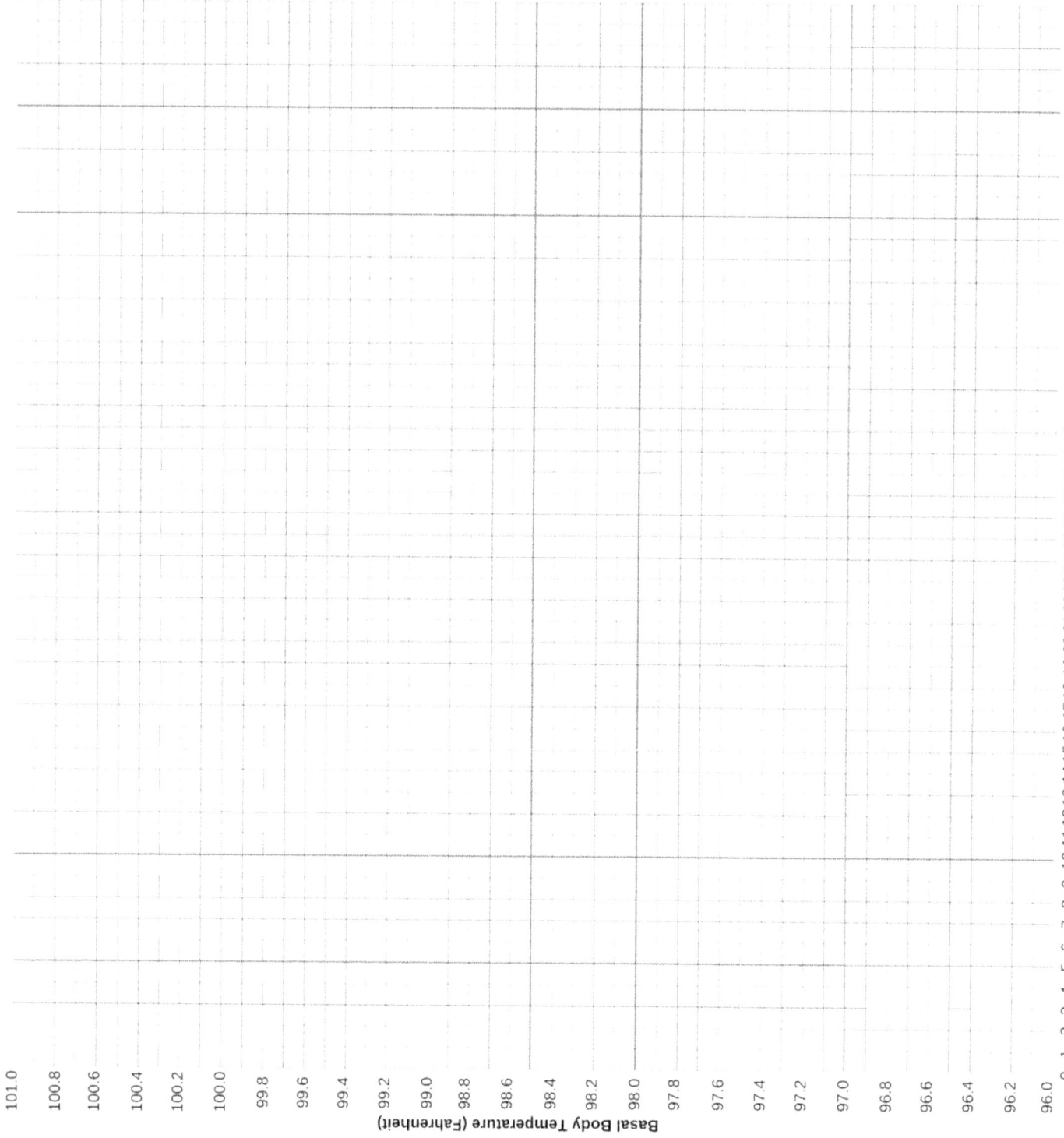

0 1 2 3 4 5 6 7 8 9 10 11 12 13 14 15 16 17 18 19 20 21 22 23 24 25 26 27 28 29 30 31 32 33 34 35 36 37 38 39 40 41 42 43 44 45 46 47 48 49 50

Day in Cycle

Cycle tracker

first day of period _____

cycle number _____

March

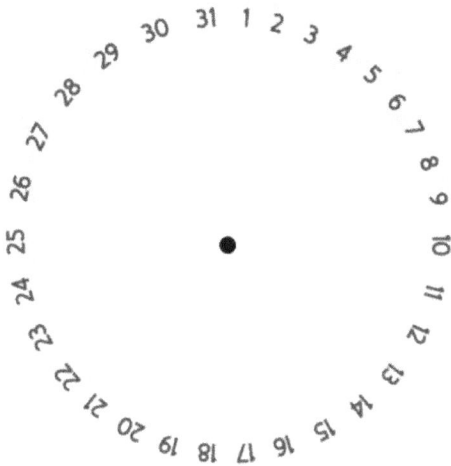

Menstruation Flow

Day 1	Day 2	Day 3
⬦⬦⬦⬦⬦	⬦⬦⬦⬦⬦	⬦⬦⬦⬦⬦

Day 4	Day 5	Day 6
⬦⬦⬦⬦⬦	⬦⬦⬦⬦⬦	⬦⬦⬦⬦⬦

Day 7
⬦⬦⬦⬦⬦

Mood

Day 1	Day 2	Day 3	Day 4	Day 5	Day 6	Day 7
calm	calm	calm	calm	calm	calm	calm
happy	happy	happy	happy	happy	happy	happy
energetic	energetic	energetic	energetic	energetic	energetic	energetic
irritated	irritated	irritated	irritated	irritated	irritated	irritated
sad	sad	sad	sad	sad	sad	sad
anxious	anxious	anxious	anxious	anxious	anxious	anxious

Symptoms

Day 1	Day 2	Day 3	Day 4	Day 5	Day 6	Day 7
acne	acne	acne	acne	acne	acne	acne
nausea	nausea	nausea	nausea	nausea	nausea	nausea
cramps	cramps	cramps	cramps	cramps	cramps	cramps
headache	headache	headache	headache	headache	headache	headache
fatigue	fatigue	fatigue	fatigue	fatigue	fatigue	fatigue
bloating	bloating	bloating	bloating	bloating	bloating	bloating
back ache	back ache	back ache	back ache	back ache	back ache	back ache
sore boobs	sore boobs	sore boobs	sore boobs	sore boobs	sore boobs	sore boobs

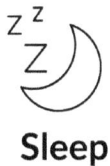

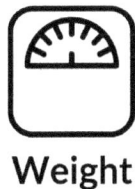

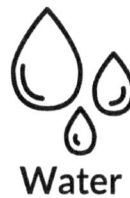

Sleep

Weight

Water

1	
2	
3	
4	
5	
6	
7	
8	
9	
10	
11	
12	
13	
14	
15	
16	
17	
18	
19	
20	
21	
22	
23	
24	
25	
26	
27	
28	
29	
30	
31	

Notes:

Daily Cycle Log

Date _____   Cycle Day _____

temperature _____   opk result _____   cervical fluid _____
(none, sticky, egg white, watery, unusual)

my mood today is...

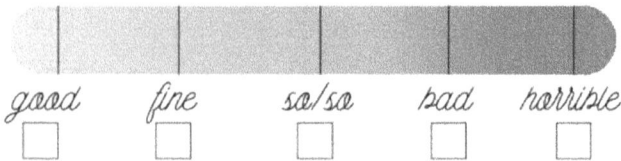

good   *fine*   *so/so*   *bad*   *horrible*
☐   ☐   ☐   ☐   ☐

thoughts about how i'm feeling :

_____

_____

_____

_____

water intake tracker

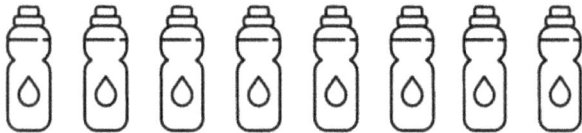

exercise

_____

meals for the day

prenatal vitamin 🗒

breakfast _____

lunch _____

dinner _____

snacks _____

Intercourse

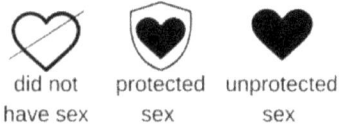

did not have sex   protected sex   unprotected sex

Mood

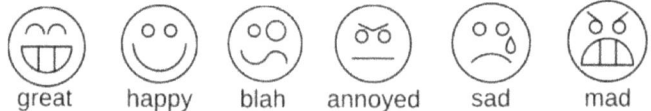

great   happy   blah   annoyed   sad   mad

Symptoms

tender breasts	headache	backache	fatigue	cravings
cramps	acne	nausea	bloating	insomnia
constipation	diarrhea	joint pain	spotting	congestion

Date _____ # Daily Cycle Log Cycle Day_____

temperature _____   opk result_____   cervical fluid _____
(none, sticky, egg white, watery, unusual)

my mood today is...

good   fine   so/so   bad   horrible
☐   ☐   ☐   ☐   ☐

water intake tracker

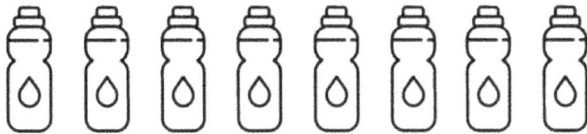

meals for the day

breakfast _____

lunch _____

dinner _____

snacks _____

thoughts about how i'm feeling :

_____

_____

_____

_____

exercise

prenatal vitamin ▢

Intercourse

did not have sex   protected sex   unprotected sex

Mood

great   happy   blah   annoyed   sad   mad

Symptoms

tender breasts	headache	backache	fatigue	cravings
cramps	acne	nausea	bloating	insomnia
constipation	diarrhea	joint pain	spotting	congestion

Daily Cycle Log

Date _____   Cycle Day_____

temperature _____   opk result _____   cervical fluid _____
(none, sticky, egg white, watery, unusual)

my mood today is...

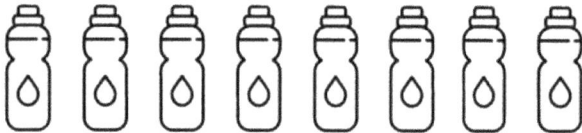

good   fine   so/so   bad   horrible
☐   ☐   ☐   ☐   ☐

thoughts about how i'm feeling :

_____

_____

_____

_____

water intake tracker

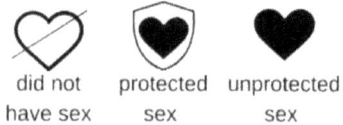

exercise
```
┌─────────────────────────────┐
│                             │
│                             │
│                             │
└─────────────────────────────┘
```

meals for the day

prenatal vitamin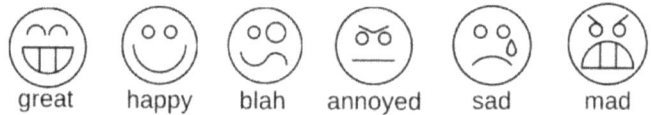

breakfast_____

lunch_____

dinner_____

snacks_____

Intercourse

did not have sex   protected sex   unprotected sex

Mood

great   happy   blah   annoyed   sad   mad

Symptoms

tender breasts	headache	backache	fatigue	cravings
cramps	acne	nausea	bloating	insomnia
constipation	diarrhea	joint pain	spotting	congestion

Daily Cycle Log

Date _____   Cycle Day _____

temperature _____   opk result _____   cervical fluid _____
(none, sticky, egg white, watery, unusual)

my mood today is...

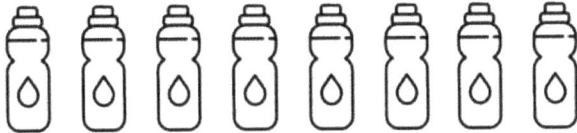

good	fine	so/so	bad	horrible
☐	☐	☐	☐	☐

thoughts about how i'm feeling :

_____
_____
_____
_____

water intake tracker

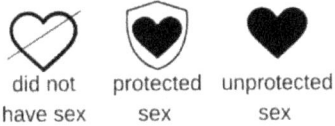

exercise

meals for the day

prenatal vitamin 📑

*breakfast*_____

*lunch*_____

*dinner*_____

*snacks*_____

Intercourse

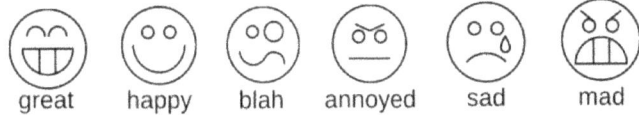

did not have sex   protected sex   unprotected sex

Mood

great   happy   blah   annoyed   sad   mad

Symptoms

tender breasts	headache	backache	fatigue	cravings
cramps	acne	nausea	bloating	insomnia
constipation	diarrhea	joint pain	spotting	congestion

Date _____   # Daily Cycle Log   Cycle Day_____

temperature _____   opk result _____   cervical fluid _____
(none, sticky, egg white, watery, unusual)

my mood today is...

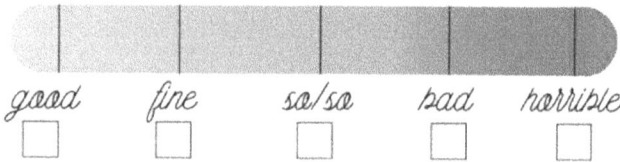

good   fine   so/so   bad   horrible
☐   ☐   ☐   ☐   ☐

thoughts about how i'm feeling :

_____

_____

_____

_____

water intake tracker

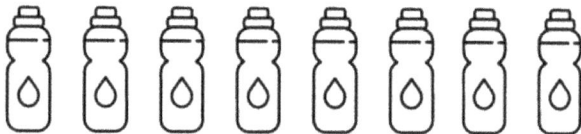

```
exercise



```

meals for the day

prenatal vitamin ▢

breakfast_____

lunch_____

dinner_____

snacks_____

Intercourse

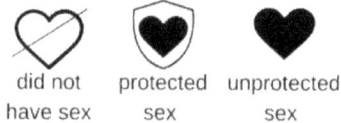

did not   protected   unprotected
have sex   sex   sex

Mood

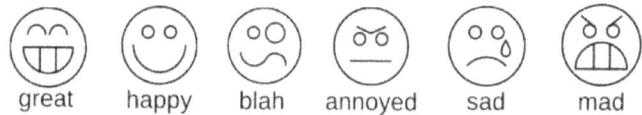

great   happy   blah   annoyed   sad   mad

Symptoms

tender breasts	headache	backache	fatigue	cravings
cramps	acne	nausea	bloating	insomnia
constipation	diarrhea	joint pain	spotting	congestion

Date _____ # Daily Cycle Log Cycle Day_____

temperature _____   opk result_____   cervical fluid _____
(none, sticky, egg white, watery, unusual)

my mood today is...

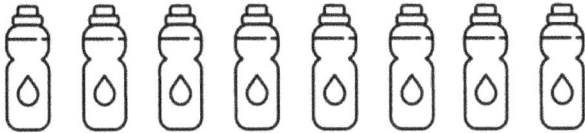

good *fine* *so/so* *bad* *horrible*
☐   ☐   ☐   ☐   ☐

thoughts about how i'm feeling :

_____

_____

_____

_____

water intake tracker

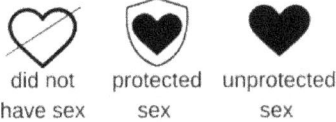

exercise

meals for the day

prenatal vitamin ☑

*breakfast*_____

lunch _____

*dinner*_____

snacks _____

Intercourse

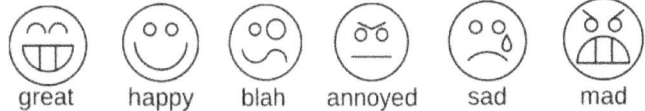

did not   protected   unprotected
have sex   sex   sex

Mood

great   happy   blah   annoyed   sad   mad

Symptoms

tender breasts	headache	backache	fatigue	cravings
cramps	acne	nausea	bloating	insomnia
constipation	diarrhea	joint pain	spotting	congestion

Daily Cycle Log

Date _____   Cycle Day _____

temperature _____   opk result _____   cervical fluid _____
(none, sticky, egg white, watery, unusual)

my mood today is...

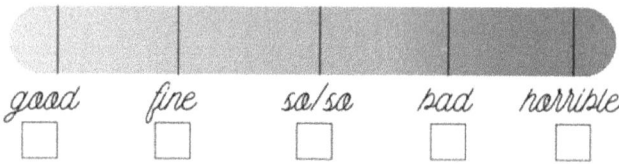

good   fine   so/so   bad   horrible
☐   ☐   ☐   ☐   ☐

thoughts about how i'm feeling :

_____
_____
_____
_____

water intake tracker

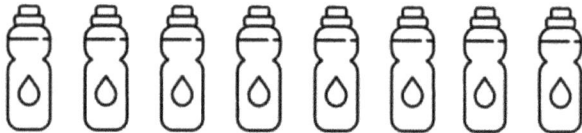

exercise
_____

meals for the day

prenatal vitamin 🔲

breakfast _____

lunch _____

dinner _____

snacks _____

Intercourse

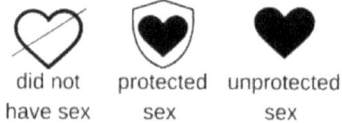

did not have sex   protected sex   unprotected sex

Mood

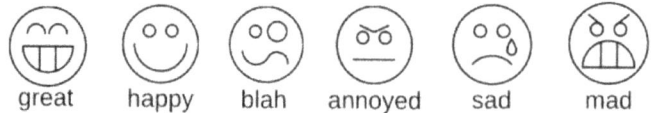

great   happy   blah   annoyed   sad   mad

Symptoms

tender breasts	headache	backache	fatigue	cravings
cramps	acne	nausea	bloating	insomnia
constipation	diarrhea	joint pain	spotting	congestion

basal body Temperature chart

Basal Body Temperature (Fahrenheit)

101.0
100.8
100.6
100.4
100.2
100.0
99.8
99.6
99.4
99.2
99.0
98.8
98.6
98.4
98.2
98.0
97.8
97.6
97.4
97.2
97.0
96.8
96.6
96.4
96.2
96.0

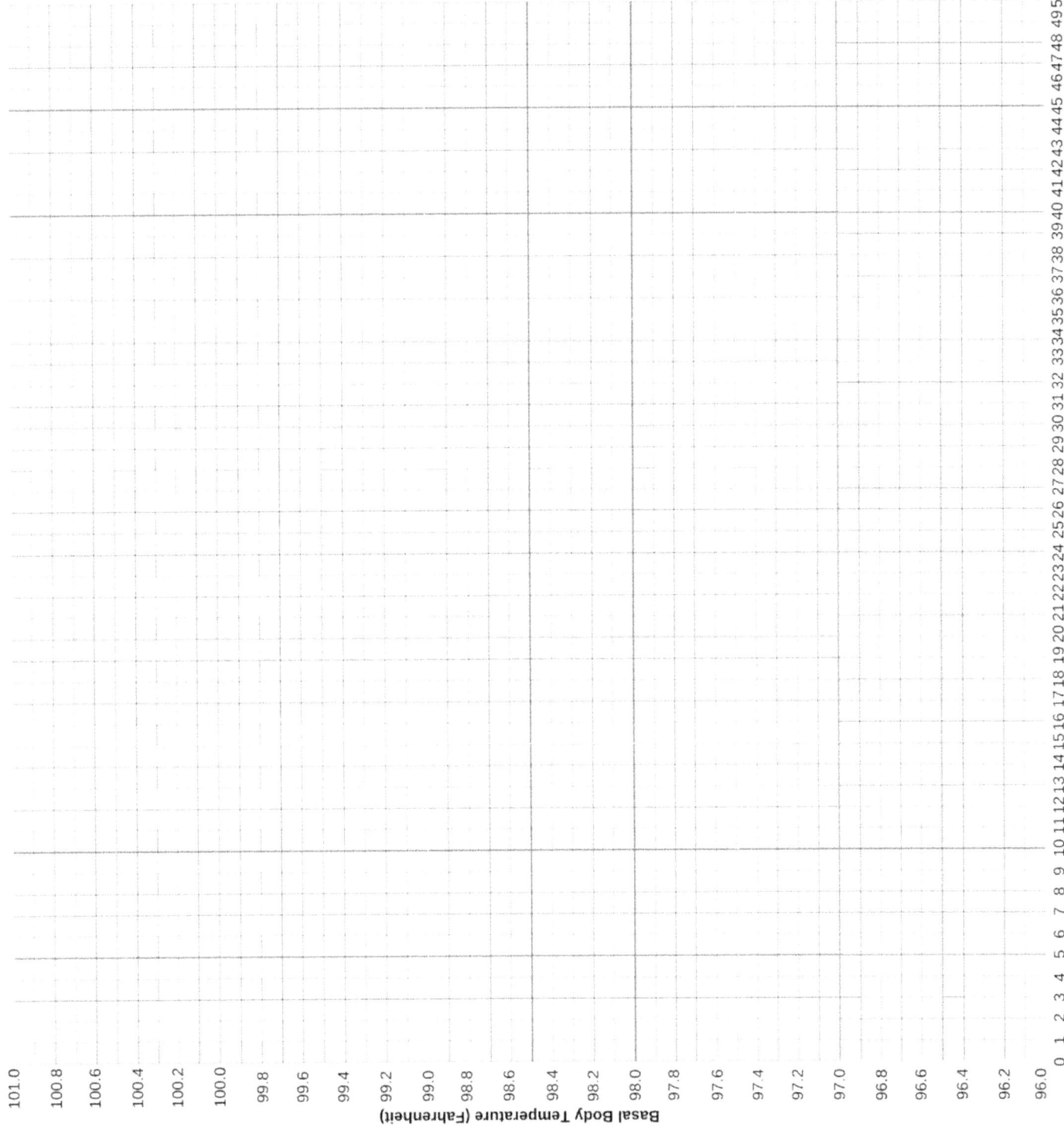

0 1 2 3 4 5 6 7 8 9 10 11 12 13 14 15 16 17 18 19 20 21 22 23 24 25 26 27 28 29 30 31 32 33 34 35 36 37 38 39 40 41 42 43 44 45 46 47 48 49 50

Day in Cycle

Cycle tracker

first day of period _____

cycle number _____

April

Menstruation Flow

Day 1	Day 2	Day 3
⬡⬡⬡⬡⬡	⬡⬡⬡⬡⬡	⬡⬡⬡⬡⬡

Day 4	Day 5	Day 6
⬡⬡⬡⬡⬡	⬡⬡⬡⬡⬡	⬡⬡⬡⬡⬡

Day 7

⬡⬡⬡⬡⬡

Mood

Day 1	Day 2	Day 3	Day 4	Day 5	Day 6	Day 7
calm	calm	calm	calm	calm	calm	calm
happy	happy	happy	happy	happy	happy	happy
energetic	energetic	energetic	energetic	energetic	energetic	energetic
irritated	irritated	irritated	irritated	irritated	irritated	irritated
sad	sad	sad	sad	sad	sad	sad
anxious	anxious	anxious	anxious	anxious	anxious	anxious

Symptoms

Day 1	Day 2	Day 3	Day 4	Day 5	Day 6	Day 7
acne	acne	acne	acne	acne	acne	acne
nausea	nausea	nausea	nausea	nausea	nausea	nausea
cramps	cramps	cramps	cramps	cramps	cramps	cramps
headache	headache	headache	headache	headache	headache	headache
fatigue	fatigue	fatigue	fatigue	fatigue	fatigue	fatigue
bloating	bloating	bloating	bloating	bloating	bloating	bloating
back ache	back ache	back ache	back ache	back ache	back ache	back ache
sore boobs	sore boobs	sore boobs	sore boobs	sore boobs	sore boobs	sore boobs

Sleep

Weight

Water

1	
2	
3	
4	
5	
6	
7	
8	
9	
10	
11	
12	
13	
14	
15	
16	
17	
18	
19	
20	
21	
22	
23	
24	
25	
26	
27	
28	
29	
30	
31	

Notes:

Date _____ **Daily Cycle Log** Cycle Day_____

temperature _____ opk result _____ cervical fluid _____
(none, sticky, egg white, watery, unusual)

my mood today is...

good | fine | so/so | bad | horrible
☐ | ☐ | ☐ | ☐ | ☐

thoughts about how i'm feeling :

_____
_____
_____
_____

water intake tracker

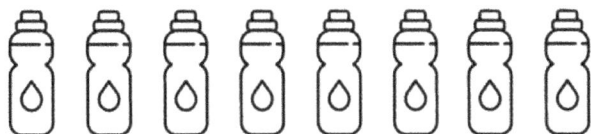

exercise

meals for the day

prenatal vitamin ☐

breakfast_____

lunch_____

dinner_____

snacks_____

Intercourse

did not have sex | protected sex | unprotected sex

Mood

great | happy | blah | annoyed | sad | mad

Symptoms

tender breasts	headache	backache	fatigue	cravings
cramps	acne	nausea	bloating	insomnia
constipation	diarrhea	joint pain	spotting	congestion

Daily Cycle Log

Date _____   Cycle Day _____

temperature _____   opk result _____   cervical fluid _____
(none, sticky, egg white, watery, unusual)

my mood today is...

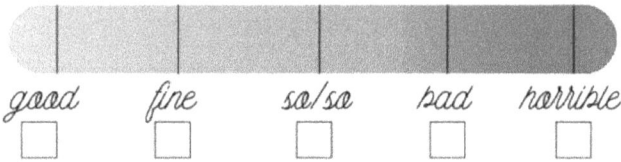

good   *fine*   *so/so*   *bad*   *horrible*
☐   ☐   ☐   ☐   ☐

thoughts about how i'm feeling :

_____
_____
_____
_____

water intake tracker

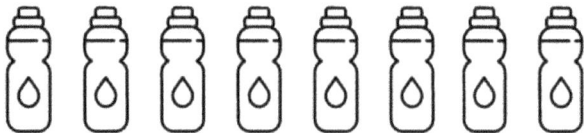

exercise
┌─────────────────────────────┐
│   │
│   │
│   │
└─────────────────────────────┘

meals for the day   prenatal vitamin ▢

breakfast _____

lunch _____

dinner _____

snacks _____

Intercourse

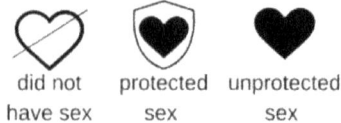

did not   protected   unprotected
have sex   sex   sex

Mood

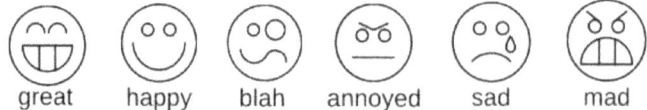

great   happy   blah   annoyed   sad   mad

Symptoms

tender breasts   headache   backache   fatigue   cravings

cramps   acne   nausea   bloating   insomnia

constipation   diarrhea   joint pain   spotting   congestion

Date _____ # Daily Cycle Log Cycle Day_____

temperature _____ opk result _____ cervical fluid _____
(none, sticky, egg white, watery, unusual)

my mood today is...

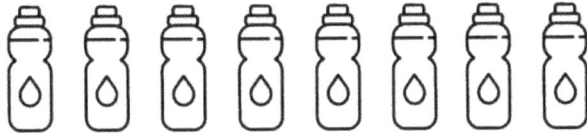

good   fine   so/so   bad   horrible
☐   ☐   ☐   ☐   ☐

water intake tracker

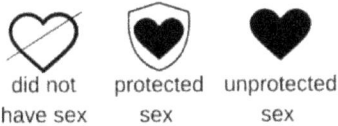

thoughts about how i'm feeling :

_____

_____

_____

_____

exercise

prenatal vitamin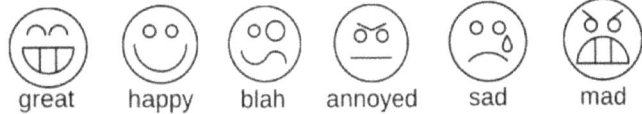

meals for the day

breakfast_____

lunch_____

dinner_____

snacks_____

Intercourse

♡   🛡   ♥
did not   protected   unprotected
have sex   sex   sex

Mood

great   happy   blah   annoyed   sad   mad

Symptoms

tender breasts	headache	backache	fatigue	cravings
cramps	acne	nausea	bloating	insomnia
constipation	diarrhea	joint pain	spotting	congestion

Daily Cycle Log

Date _____   Cycle Day _____

temperature _____   opk result _____   cervical fluid _____
(none, sticky, egg white, watery, unusual)

my mood today is...

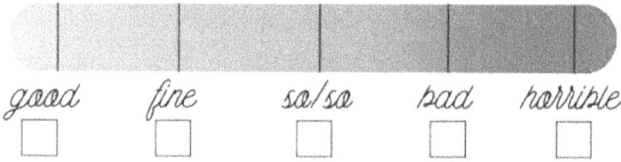

good   *fine*   *so/so*   *bad*   *horrible*
☐   ☐   ☐   ☐   ☐

thoughts about how i'm feeling :

_____
_____
_____
_____

water intake tracker

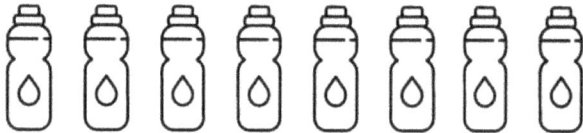

exercise
_____

meals for the day

prenatal vitamin

breakfast _____

lunch _____

dinner _____

snacks _____

Intercourse

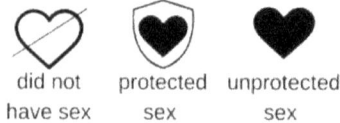

did not   protected   unprotected
have sex   sex   sex

Mood

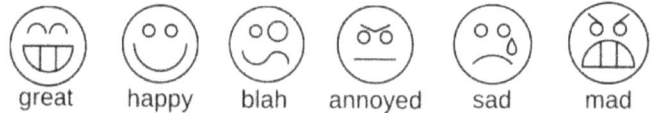

great   happy   blah   annoyed   sad   mad

Symptoms

tender breasts	headache	backache	fatigue	cravings
cramps	acne	nausea	bloating	insomnia
constipation	diarrhea	joint pain	spotting	congestion

Date _____ # Daily Cycle Log Cycle Day _____

temperature _____   opk result _____   cervical fluid _____
(none, sticky, egg white, watery, unusual)

my mood today is...

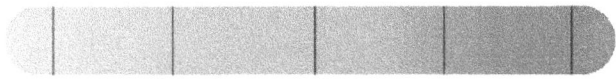

good   fine   so/so   bad   horrible
☐   ☐   ☐   ☐   ☐

thoughts about how i'm feeling :

_____

_____

_____

_____

water intake tracker

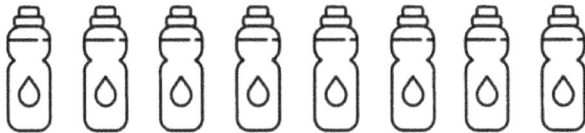

exercise

meals for the day

prenatal vitamin ☐

breakfast _____

lunch _____

dinner _____

snacks _____

Intercourse

did not have sex   protected sex   unprotected sex

Mood

great   happy   blah   annoyed   sad   mad

Symptoms

tender breasts	headache	backache	fatigue	cravings
cramps	acne	nausea	bloating	insomnia
constipation	diarrhea	joint pain	spotting	congestion

Daily Cycle Log

Date _____   Cycle Day _____

temperature _____   opk result _____   cervical fluid _____
(none, sticky, egg white, watery, unusual)

my mood today is...

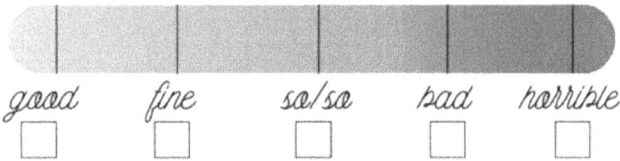

good   *fine*   *so/so*   *bad*   *horrible*
☐   ☐   ☐   ☐   ☐

thoughts about how i'm feeling :

_____
_____
_____
_____

water intake tracker

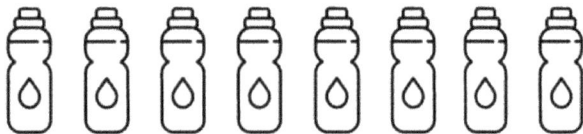

exercise

_____

meals for the day

prenatal vitamin ▢

breakfast _____

lunch _____

dinner _____

snacks _____

Intercourse

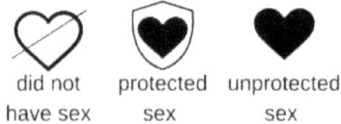

did not have sex   protected sex   unprotected sex

Mood

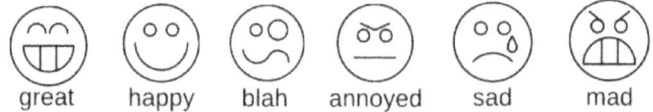

great   happy   blah   annoyed   sad   mad

Symptoms

tender breasts	headache	backache	fatigue	cravings
cramps	acne	nausea	bloating	insomnia
constipation	diarrhea	joint pain	spotting	congestion

Date _____   # Daily Cycle Log   Cycle Day _____

temperature _____   opk result _____   cervical fluid _____
(none, sticky, egg white, watery, unusual)

my mood today is...

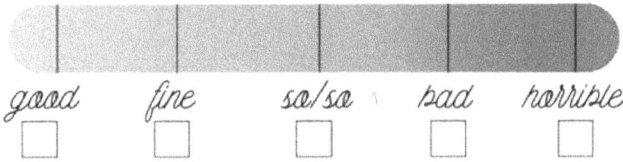

good   fine   so/so   bad   horrible
☐   ☐   ☐   ☐   ☐

thoughts about how i'm feeling :

_____

_____

_____

_____

water intake tracker

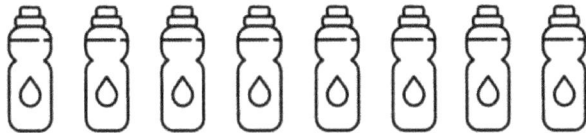

exercise

meals for the day

prenatal vitamin 🗒

breakfast _____

lunch _____

dinner _____

snacks _____

Intercourse

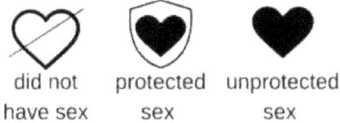

did not have sex   protected sex   unprotected sex

Mood

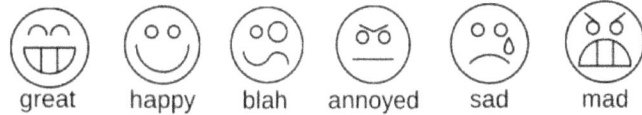

great   happy   blah   annoyed   sad   mad

Symptoms

tender breasts	headache	backache	fatigue	cravings
cramps	acne	nausea	bloating	insomnia
constipation	diarrhea	joint pain	spotting	congestion

date range _____

basal body Temperature Chart

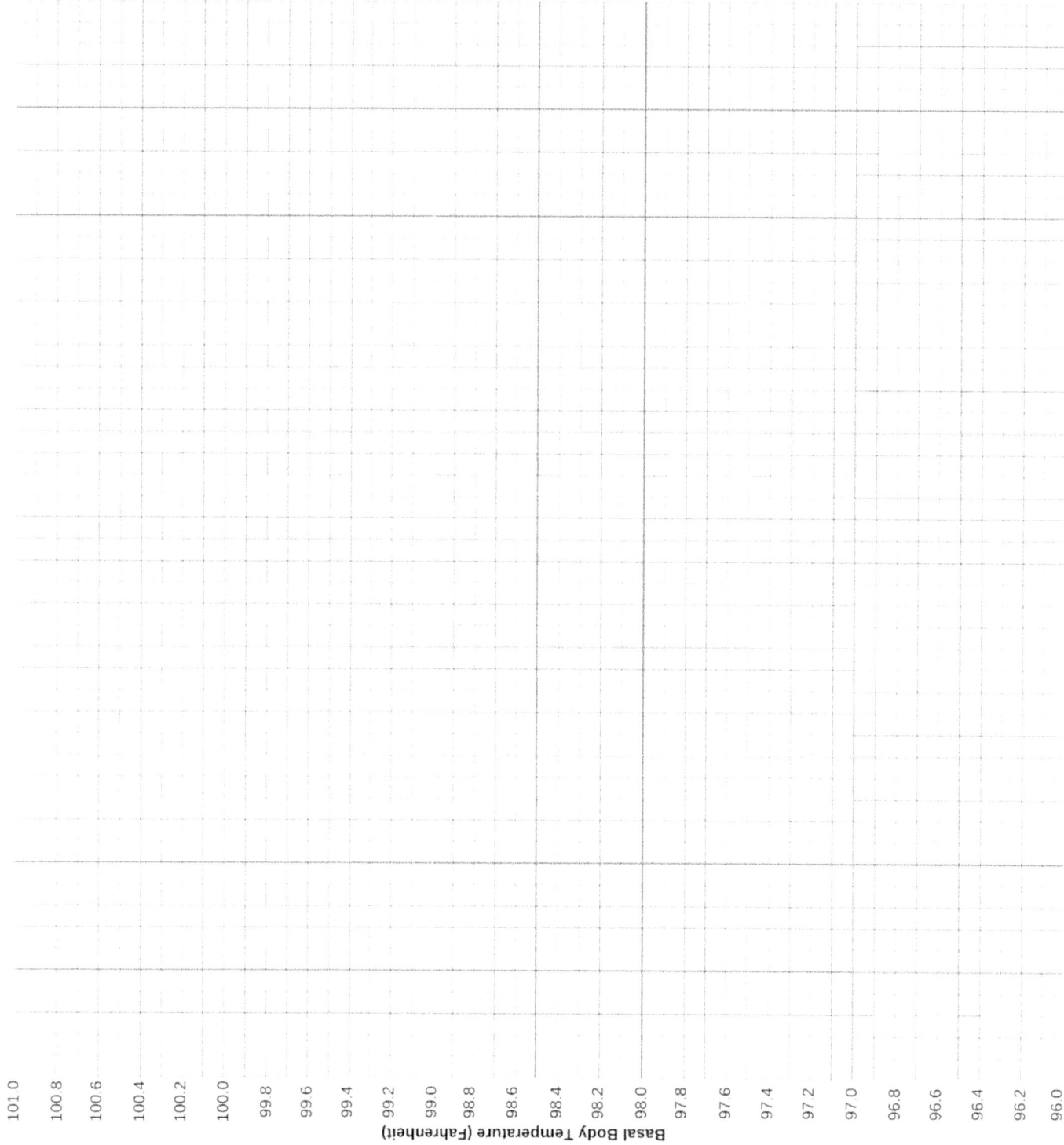

cycle # _____

Basal Body Temperature (Fahrenheit)

101.0
100.8
100.6
100.4
100.2
100.0
99.8
99.6
99.4
99.2
99.0
98.8
98.6
98.4
98.2
98.0
97.8
97.6
97.4
97.2
97.0
96.8
96.6
96.4
96.2
96.0

0 1 2 3 4 5 6 7 8 9 10 11 12 13 14 15 16 17 18 19 20 21 22 23 24 25 26 27 28 29 30 31 32 33 34 35 36 37 38 39 40 41 42 43 44 45 46 47 48 49 50

Day in Cycle

Cycle tracker

first day of period _____

cycle number _____

May

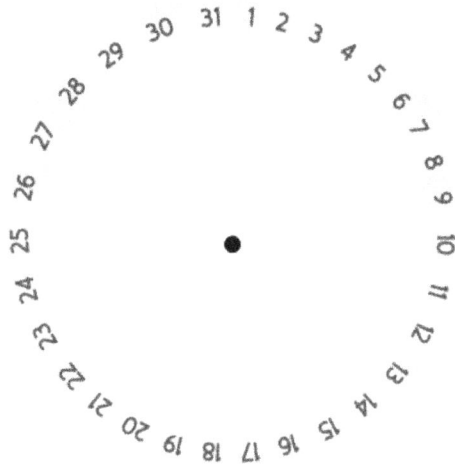

Menstruation Flow

Day 1	Day 2	Day 3
⬡⬡⬡⬡⬡	⬡⬡⬡⬡⬡	⬡⬡⬡⬡⬡

Day 4	Day 5	Day 6
⬡⬡⬡⬡⬡	⬡⬡⬡⬡⬡	⬡⬡⬡⬡⬡

Day 7

⬡⬡⬡⬡⬡

Mood

Day 1	Day 2	Day 3	Day 4	Day 5	Day 6	Day 7
calm	calm	calm	calm	calm	calm	calm
happy	happy	happy	happy	happy	happy	happy
energetic	energetic	energetic	energetic	energetic	energetic	energetic
irritated	irritated	irritated	irritated	irritated	irritated	irritated
sad	sad	sad	sad	sad	sad	sad
anxious	anxious	anxious	anxious	anxious	anxious	anxious

Symptoms

Day 1	Day 2	Day 3	Day 4	Day 5	Day 6	Day 7
acne	acne	acne	acne	acne	acne	acne
nausea	nausea	nausea	nausea	nausea	nausea	nausea
cramps	cramps	cramps	cramps	cramps	cramps	cramps
headache	headache	headache	headache	headache	headache	headache
fatigue	fatigue	fatigue	fatigue	fatigue	fatigue	fatigue
bloating	bloating	bloating	bloating	bloating	bloating	bloating
back ache	back ache	back ache	back ache	back ache	back ache	back ache
sore boobs	sore boobs	sore boobs	sore boobs	sore boobs	sore boobs	sore boobs

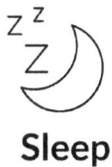

Sleep

_____

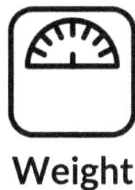

Weight

_____

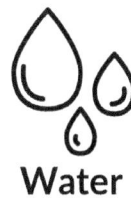

Water

_____

1	
2	
3	
4	
5	
6	
7	
8	
9	
10	
11	
12	
13	
14	
15	
16	
17	
18	
19	
20	
21	
22	
23	
24	
25	
26	
27	
28	
29	
30	
31	

Notes:

Date _____ # Daily Cycle Log Cycle Day _____

temperature _____ opk result _____ cervical fluid _____
(none, sticky, egg white, watery, unusual)

my mood today is...

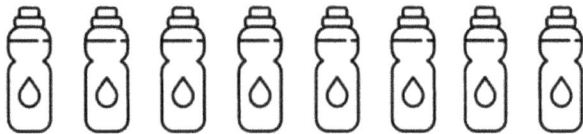

good   fine   so/so   bad   horrible
☐   ☐   ☐   ☐   ☐

thoughts about how i'm feeling :

_____

_____

_____

_____

water intake tracker

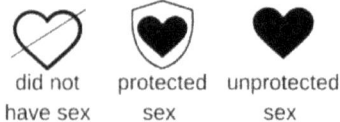

exercise

meals for the day

prenatal vitamin ◻

breakfast _____

lunch _____

dinner _____

snacks _____

Intercourse

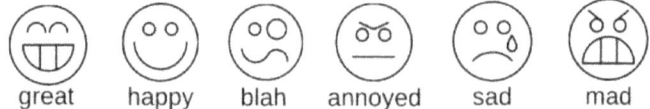

did not have sex   protected sex   unprotected sex

Mood

great   happy   blah   annoyed   sad   mad

Symptoms

tender breasts	headache	backache	fatigue	cravings
cramps	acne	nausea	bloating	insomnia
constipation	diarrhea	joint pain	spotting	congestion

Daily Cycle Log

Date _____ Cycle Day _____

temperature _____ opk result _____ cervical fluid _____
(none, sticky, egg white, watery, unusual)

my mood today is...

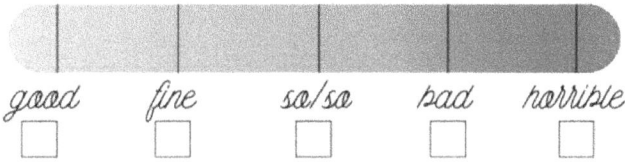

good   fine   so/so   bad   horrible
☐   ☐   ☐   ☐   ☐

water intake tracker

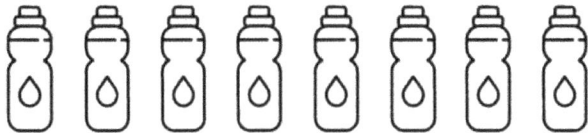

thoughts about how i'm feeling :

_____

_____

_____

_____

exercise
[   ]

meals for the day

prenatal vitamin ☐

breakfast _____

lunch _____

dinner _____

snacks _____

Intercourse

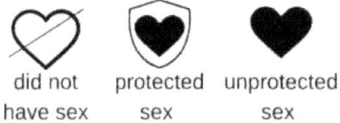

did not have sex   protected sex   unprotected sex

Mood

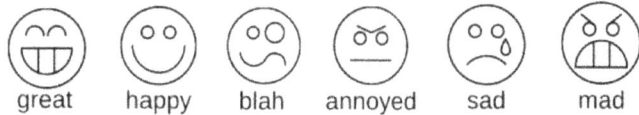

great   happy   blah   annoyed   sad   mad

Symptoms

tender breasts	headache	backache	fatigue	cravings
cramps	acne	nausea	bloating	insomnia
constipation	diarrhea	joint pain	spotting	congestion

Daily Cycle Log

Date _____   Cycle Day _____

temperature _____   opk result _____   cervical fluid _____
(none, sticky, egg white, watery, unusual)

my mood today is...

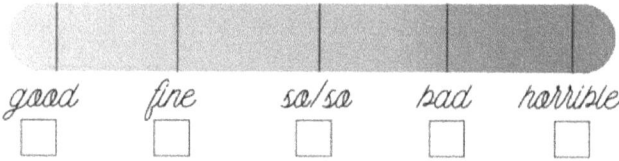

good *fine* *so/so* *bad* *horrible*
☐   ☐   ☐   ☐   ☐

thoughts about how i'm feeling :

_____
_____
_____
_____

water intake tracker

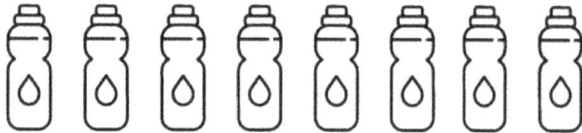

exercise
_____

meals for the day

prenatal vitamin 📖

breakfast _____

lunch _____

dinner _____

snacks _____

Intercourse

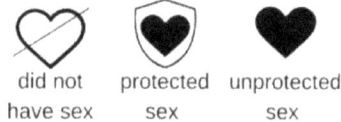

did not have sex   protected sex   unprotected sex

Mood

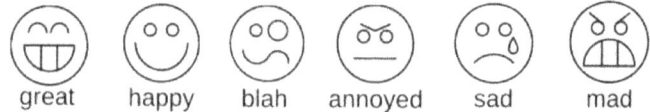

great   happy   blah   annoyed   sad   mad

Symptoms

tender breasts	headache	backache	fatigue	cravings
cramps	acne	nausea	bloating	insomnia
constipation	diarrhea	joint pain	spotting	congestion

Daily Cycle Log

Date _____   Cycle Day _____

temperature _____   opk result _____   cervical fluid _____
(none, sticky, egg white, watery, unusual)

my mood today is...

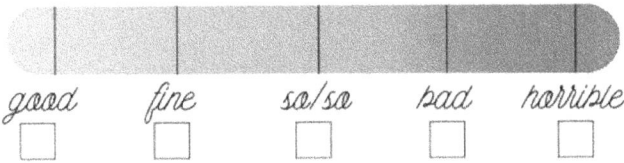

good   fine   so/so   bad   horrible
☐   ☐   ☐   ☐   ☐

water intake tracker

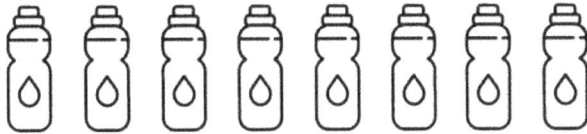

thoughts about how i'm feeling :

_____
_____
_____
_____

exercise

prenatal vitamin ⧉

meals for the day

breakfast _____

lunch _____

dinner _____

snacks _____

Intercourse

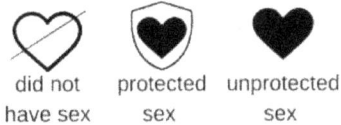

did not have sex   protected sex   unprotected sex

Mood

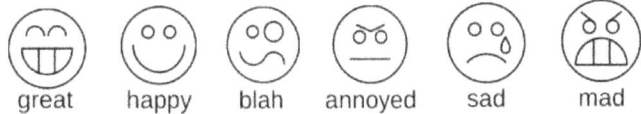

great   happy   blah   annoyed   sad   mad

Symptoms

tender breasts	headache	backache	fatigue	cravings
cramps	acne	nausea	bloating	insomnia
constipation	diarrhea	joint pain	spotting	congestion

Daily Cycle Log

Date _____

Cycle Day _____

temperature _____

opk result _____

cervical fluid _____
(none, sticky, egg white, watery, unusual)

my mood today is...

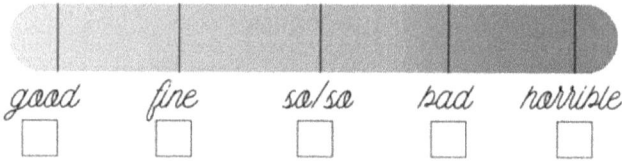

good   fine   so/so   bad   horrible
☐   ☐   ☐   ☐   ☐

thoughts about how i'm feeling :

_____
_____
_____
_____

water intake tracker

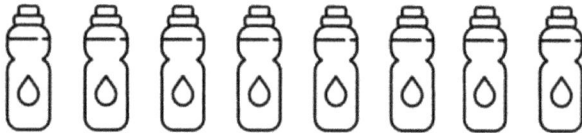

exercise
_____

meals for the day

prenatal vitamin ▢

breakfast _____

lunch _____

dinner _____

snacks _____

Intercourse

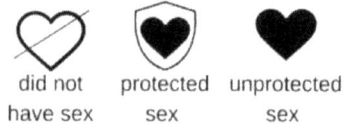

did not   protected   unprotected
have sex   sex   sex

Mood

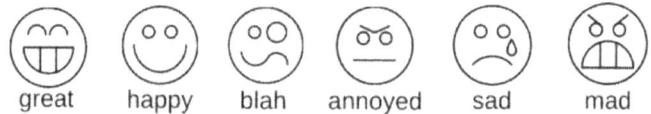

great   happy   blah   annoyed   sad   mad

Symptoms

tender breasts	headache	backache	fatigue	cravings
cramps	acne	nausea	bloating	insomnia
constipation	diarrhea	joint pain	spotting	congestion

Daily Cycle Log

Date _____   Cycle Day _____

temperature _____   opk result _____   cervical fluid _____
(none, sticky, egg white, watery, unusual)

my mood today is...

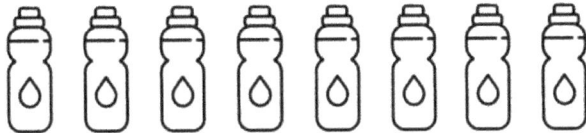

good   fine   so/so   bad   horrible
☐   ☐   ☐   ☐   ☐

thoughts about how i'm feeling :

_____
_____
_____
_____

water intake tracker

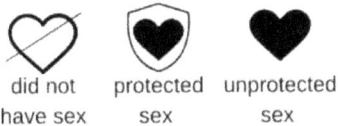

exercise

meals for the day

prenatal vitamin 🗒

breakfast _____

lunch _____

dinner _____

snacks _____

Intercourse

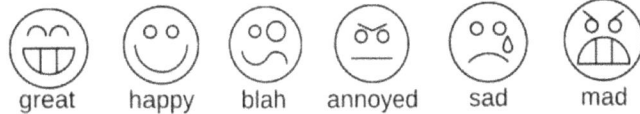

did not   protected   unprotected
have sex   sex   sex

Mood

great   happy   blah   annoyed   sad   mad

Symptoms

tender breasts	headache	backache	fatigue	cravings
cramps	acne	nausea	bloating	insomnia
constipation	diarrhea	joint pain	spotting	congestion

Date _____ **Daily Cycle Log** Cycle Day_____

temperature _____ opk result _____ cervical fluid _____
(none, sticky, egg white, watery, unusual)

my mood today is...

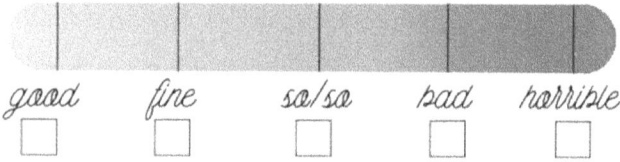

good *fine* *so/so* *bad* *horrible*
☐   ☐   ☐   ☐   ☐

water intake tracker

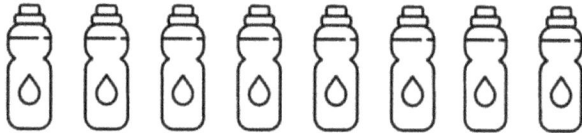

thoughts about how i'm feeling :

_____
_____
_____
_____

exercise

prenatal vitamin 📑

meals for the day

*breakfast*_____

*lunch*_____

*dinner*_____

*snacks*_____

Intercourse

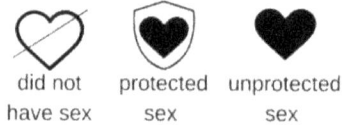

did not   protected   unprotected
have sex   sex   sex

Mood

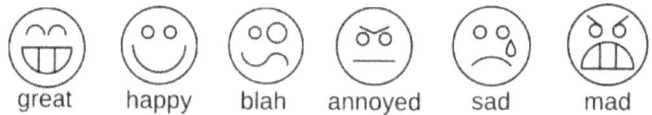

great   happy   blah   annoyed   sad   mad

Symptoms

tender breasts	headache	backache	fatigue	cravings
cramps	acne	nausea	bloating	insomnia
constipation	diarrhea	joint pain	spotting	congestion

basal body temperature chart

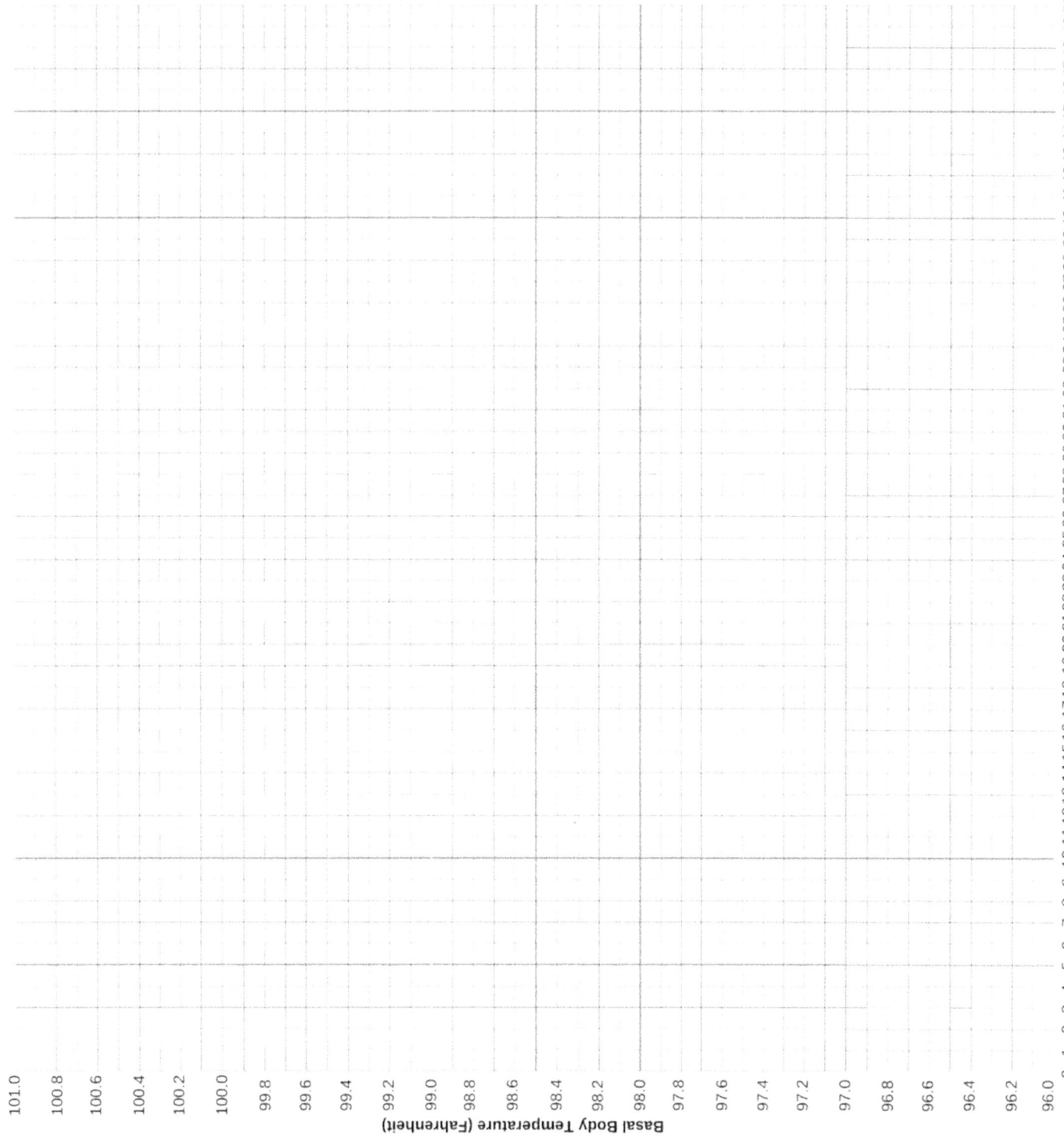

Basal Body Temperature (Fahrenheit)

101.0
100.8
100.6
100.4
100.2
100.0
99.8
99.6
99.4
99.2
99.0
98.8
98.6
98.4
98.2
98.0
97.8
97.6
97.4
97.2
97.0
96.8
96.6
96.4
96.2
96.0

0 1 2 3 4 5 6 7 8 9 10 11 12 13 14 15 16 17 18 19 20 21 22 23 24 25 26 27 28 29 30 31 32 33 34 35 36 37 38 39 40 41 42 43 44 45 46 47 48 49 50

Day in Cycle

Cycle tracker

first day of period _____

cycle number _____

June

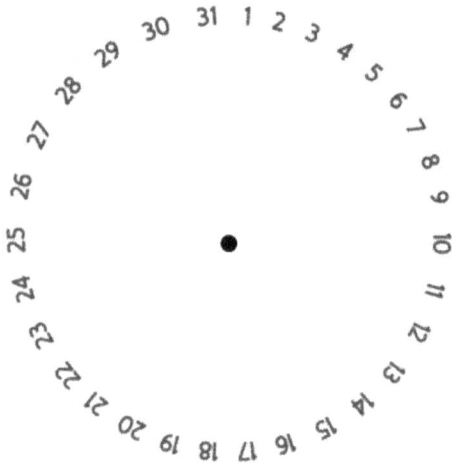

Menstruation Flow

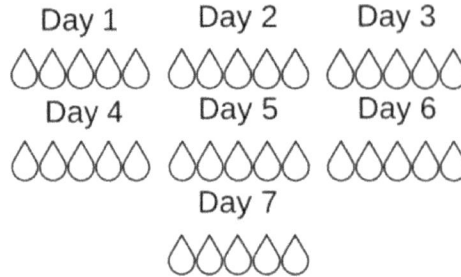

Day 1	Day 2	Day 3
⬡⬡⬡⬡⬡	⬡⬡⬡⬡⬡	⬡⬡⬡⬡⬡

Day 4	Day 5	Day 6
⬡⬡⬡⬡⬡	⬡⬡⬡⬡⬡	⬡⬡⬡⬡⬡

Day 7

⬡⬡⬡⬡⬡

Mood

Day 1	Day 2	Day 3	Day 4	Day 5	Day 6	Day 7
calm	calm	calm	calm	calm	calm	calm
happy	happy	happy	happy	happy	happy	happy
energetic	energetic	energetic	energetic	energetic	energetic	energetic
irritated	irritated	irritated	irritated	irritated	irritated	irritated
sad	sad	sad	sad	sad	sad	sad
anxious	anxious	anxious	anxious	anxious	anxious	anxious

Symptoms

Day 1	Day 2	Day 3	Day 4	Day 5	Day 6	Day 7
acne	acne	acne	acne	acne	acne	acne
nausea	nausea	nausea	nausea	nausea	nausea	nausea
cramps	cramps	cramps	cramps	cramps	cramps	cramps
headache	headache	headache	headache	headache	headache	headache
fatigue	fatigue	fatigue	fatigue	fatigue	fatigue	fatigue
bloating	bloating	bloating	bloating	bloating	bloating	bloating
back ache	back ache	back ache	back ache	back ache	back ache	back ache
sore boobs	sore boobs	sore boobs	sore boobs	sore boobs	sore boobs	sore boobs

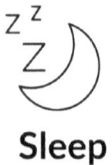

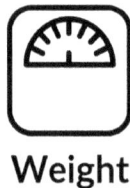

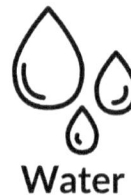

Sleep
_____

Weight
_____

Water
_____

1
2
3
4
5
6
7
8
9
10
11
12
13
14
15
16
17
18
19
20
21
22
23
24
25
26
27
28
29
30
31

Notes:

Date _____   # Daily Cycle Log   Cycle Day _____

temperature _____   opk result _____   cervical fluid _____
(none, sticky, egg white, watery, unusual)

my mood today is...

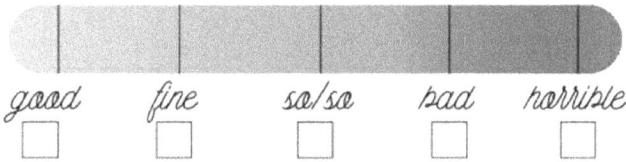

good   fine   so/so   bad   horrible
☐   ☐   ☐   ☐   ☐

thoughts about how i'm feeling :

_____

_____

_____

_____

water intake tracker

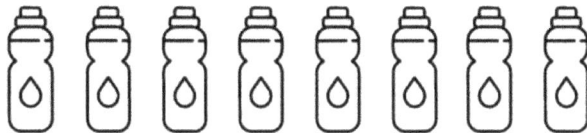

exercise

meals for the day

prenatal vitamin ⃞

breakfast _____

lunch _____

dinner _____

snacks _____

Intercourse

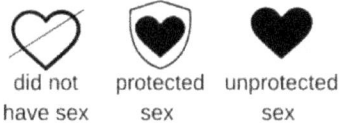

did not have sex   protected sex   unprotected sex

Mood

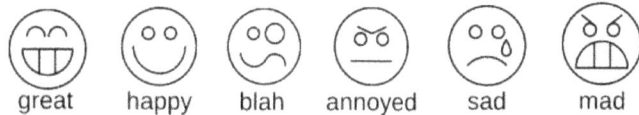

great   happy   blah   annoyed   sad   mad

Symptoms

tender breasts	headache	backache	fatigue	cravings
cramps	acne	nausea	bloating	insomnia
constipation	diarrhea	joint pain	spotting	congestion

Daily Cycle Log

Date _____   Cycle Day _____

temperature _____   opk result _____   cervical fluid _____
(none, sticky, egg white, watery, unusual)

my mood today is...

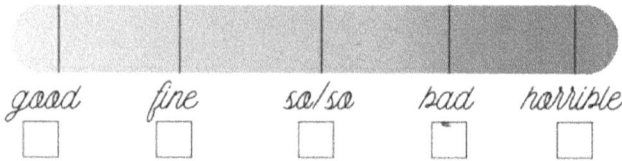

good   fine   so/so   bad   horrible
☐   ☐   ☐   ☐   ☐

water intake tracker

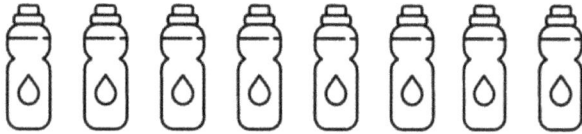

thoughts about how i'm feeling :

_____
_____
_____
_____

exercise

prenatal vitamin ▢

meals for the day

breakfast _____

lunch _____

dinner _____

snacks _____

Intercourse

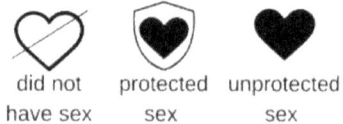

did not have sex   protected sex   unprotected sex

Mood

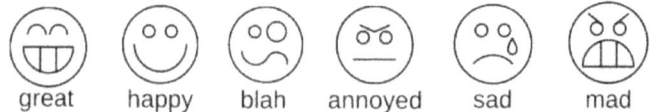

great   happy   blah   annoyed   sad   mad

Symptoms

tender breasts	headache	backache	fatigue	cravings
cramps	acne	nausea	bloating	insomnia
constipation	diarrhea	joint pain	spotting	congestion

Daily Cycle Log

Date _____   Cycle Day _____

temperature _____   opk result _____   cervical fluid _____
(none, sticky, egg white, watery, unusual)

my mood today is...

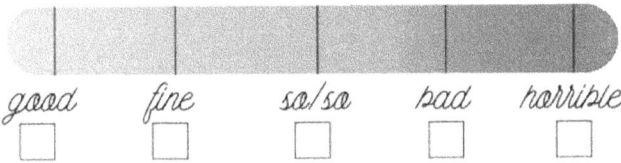

good   fine   so/so   bad   horrible
☐   ☐   ☐   ☐   ☐

water intake tracker

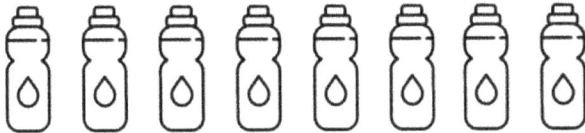

meals for the day

thoughts about how i'm feeling :

_____
_____
_____
_____

exercise
[   ]

prenatal vitamin ☐

breakfast _____
lunch _____
dinner _____
snacks _____

Intercourse

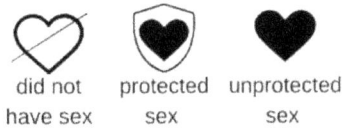

did not   protected   unprotected
have sex   sex   sex

Mood

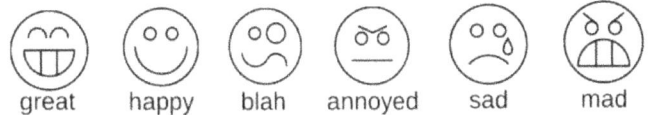

great   happy   blah   annoyed   sad   mad

Symptoms

tender breasts	headache	backache	fatigue	cravings
cramps	acne	nausea	bloating	insomnia
constipation	diarrhea	joint pain	spotting	congestion

Date _____ # Daily Cycle Log Cycle Day _____

temperature _____ opk result _____ cervical fluid _____
(none, sticky, egg white, watery, unusual)

my mood today is...

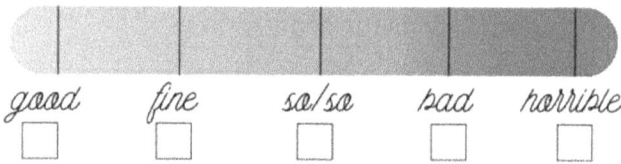

good *fine* *so/so* *bad* *horrible*
☐   ☐   ☐   ☐   ☐

water intake tracker

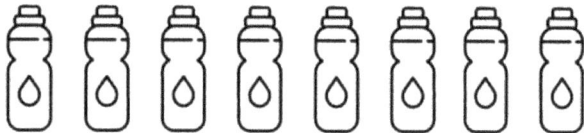

thoughts about how i'm feeling :

_____
_____
_____
_____

exercise

prenatal vitamin ▢

meals for the day

breakfast _____

lunch _____

dinner _____

snacks _____

Intercourse

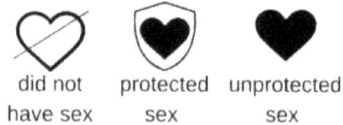

did not   protected   unprotected
have sex   sex   sex

Mood

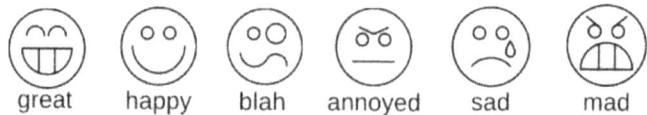

great   happy   blah   annoyed   sad   mad

Symptoms

tender breasts	headache	backache	fatigue	cravings
cramps	acne	nausea	bloating	insomnia
constipation	diarrhea	joint pain	spotting	congestion

Daily Cycle Log

Date _____ Cycle Day _____

temperature _____ opk result _____ cervical fluid _____
(none, sticky, egg white, watery, unusual)

my mood today is...

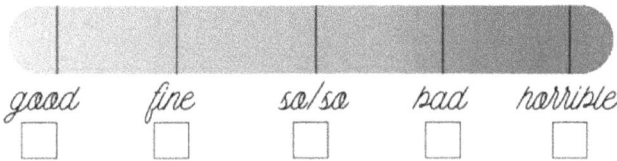

good   fine   so/so   bad   horrible
☐   ☐   ☐   ☐   ☐

thoughts about how i'm feeling :

_____

_____

_____

_____

water intake tracker

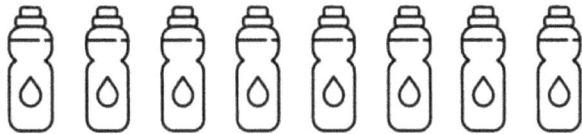

exercise

meals for the day

prenatal vitamin ❑

breakfast _____

lunch _____

dinner _____

snacks _____

Intercourse

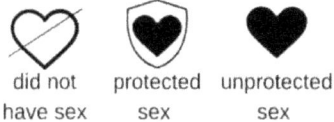

did not   protected   unprotected
have sex   sex   sex

Mood

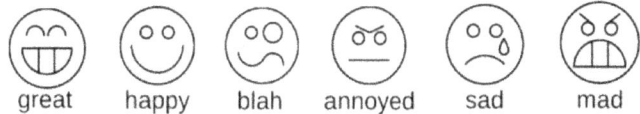

great   happy   blah   annoyed   sad   mad

Symptoms

tender breasts	headache	backache	fatigue	cravings
cramps	acne	nausea	bloating	insomnia
constipation	diarrhea	joint pain	spotting	congestion

Date _____ **Daily Cycle Log** Cycle Day_____

temperature _____   opk result_____   cervical fluid _____
(none, sticky, egg white, watery, unusual)

my mood today is...

good   *fine*   *so/so*   *bad*   *horrible*
☐   ☐   ☐   ☐   ☐

thoughts about how i'm feeling :

_____
_____
_____
_____

water intake tracker

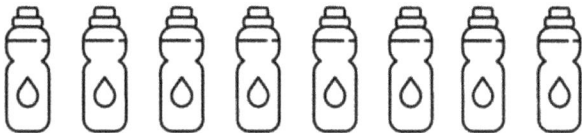

exercise

meals for the day

prenatal vitamin ▱

*breakfast*_____

*lunch*_____

*dinner*_____

*snacks*_____

Intercourse

did not have sex   protected sex   unprotected sex

Mood

great   happy   blah   annoyed   sad   mad

Symptoms

tender breasts   headache   backache   fatigue   cravings

cramps   acne   nausea   bloating   insomnia

constipation   diarrhea   joint pain   spotting   congestion

Date _____ # Daily Cycle Log Cycle Day_____

temperature _____   opk result _____   cervical fluid _____
                                                                (none, sticky, egg white, watery, unusual)

my mood today is...

good   fine   so/so   bad   horrible
☐   ☐   ☐   ☐   ☐

water intake tracker

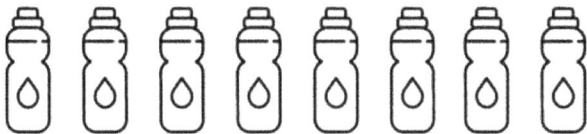

meals for the day

thoughts about how i'm feeling :

_____

_____

_____

_____

exercise

prenatal vitamin ☐

breakfast _____

lunch _____

dinner _____

snacks _____

Intercourse

did not   protected   unprotected
have sex   sex   sex

Mood

great   happy   blah   annoyed   sad   mad

Symptoms

tender breasts	headache	backache	fatigue	cravings
cramps	acne	nausea	bloating	insomnia
constipation	diarrhea	joint pain	spotting	congestion

basal body temperature chart

date range _____

cycle # _____

Basal Body Temperature (Fahrenheit)

101.0
100.8
100.6
100.4
100.2
100.0
99.8
99.6
99.4
99.2
99.0
98.8
98.6
98.4
98.2
98.0
97.8
97.6
97.4
97.2
97.0
96.8
96.6
96.4
96.2
96.0

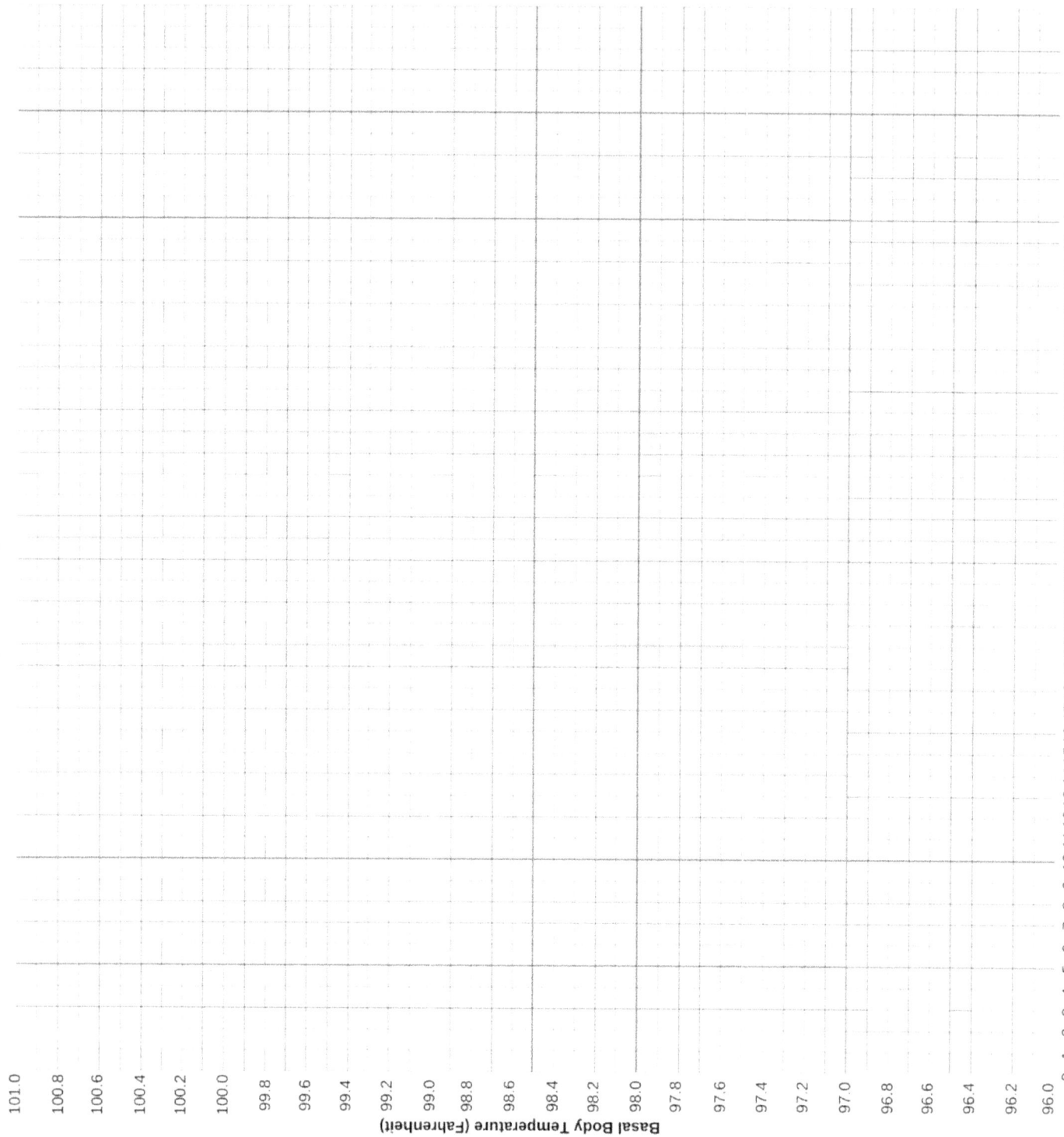

0 1 2 3 4 5 6 7 8 9 10 11 12 13 14 15 16 17 18 19 20 21 22 23 24 25 26 27 28 29 30 31 32 33 34 35 36 37 38 39 40 41 42 43 44 45 46 47 48 49 50

Day in Cycle

Cycle tracker

first day of period _____

cycle number _____

July

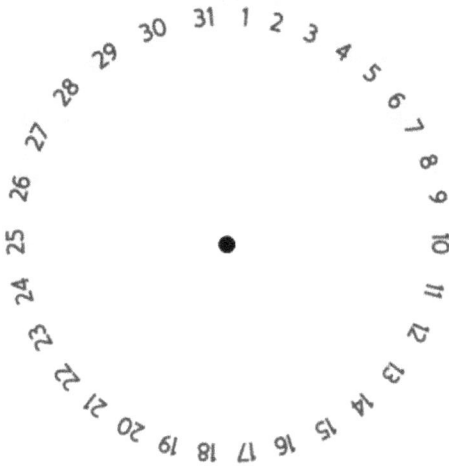

Menstruation Flow
_____

Day 1	Day 2	Day 3
⬭⬭⬭⬭⬭	⬭⬭⬭⬭⬭	⬭⬭⬭⬭⬭

Day 4	Day 5	Day 6
⬭⬭⬭⬭⬭	⬭⬭⬭⬭⬭	⬭⬭⬭⬭⬭

Day 7

⬭⬭⬭⬭⬭

Mood
_____

Day 1	Day 2	Day 3	Day 4	Day 5	Day 6	Day 7
calm	calm	calm	calm	calm	calm	calm
happy	happy	happy	happy	happy	happy	happy
energetic	energetic	energetic	energetic	energetic	energetic	energetic
irritated	irritated	irritated	irritated	irritated	irritated	irritated
sad	sad	sad	sad	sad	sad	sad
anxious	anxious	anxious	anxious	anxious	anxious	anxious

Symptoms
_____

Day 1	Day 2	Day 3	Day 4	Day 5	Day 6	Day 7
acne	acne	acne	acne	acne	acne	acne
nausea	nausea	nausea	nausea	nausea	nausea	nausea
cramps	cramps	cramps	cramps	cramps	cramps	cramps
headache	headache	headache	headache	headache	headache	headache
fatigue	fatigue	fatigue	fatigue	fatigue	fatigue	fatigue
bloating	bloating	bloating	bloating	bloating	bloating	bloating
back ache	back ache	back ache	back ache	back ache	back ache	back ache
sore boobs	sore boobs	sore boobs	sore boobs	sore boobs	sore boobs	sore boobs

Sleep

Weight

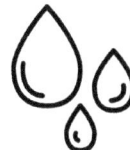

Water

1	
2	
3	
4	
5	
6	
7	
8	
9	
10	
11	
12	
13	
14	
15	
16	
17	
18	
19	
20	
21	
22	
23	
24	
25	
26	
27	
28	
29	
30	
31	

Notes:

Date _____ **Daily Cycle Log** Cycle Day_____

temperature _____   opk result _____   cervical fluid _____
(none, sticky, egg white, watery, unusual)

my mood today is...

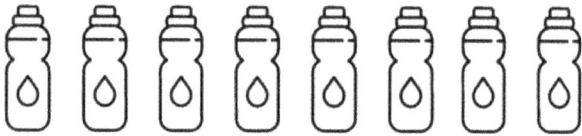

good   fine   so/so   bad   horrible
☐   ☐   ☐   ☐   ☐

thoughts about how i'm feeling :

_____
_____
_____
_____

water intake tracker

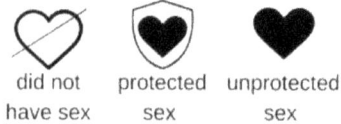

exercise

meals for the day   prenatal vitamin ▢

breakfast_____

lunch_____

dinner_____

snacks_____

Intercourse

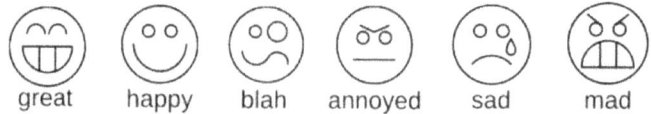

did not   protected   unprotected
have sex   sex   sex

Mood

great   happy   blah   annoyed   sad   mad

Symptoms

tender breasts   headache   backache   fatigue   cravings

cramps   acne   nausea   bloating   insomnia

constipation   diarrhea   joint pain   spotting   congestion

Daily Cycle Log

Date _____ Cycle Day_____

temperature _____ opk result _____ cervical fluid _____
(none, sticky, egg white, watery, unusual)

my mood today is...

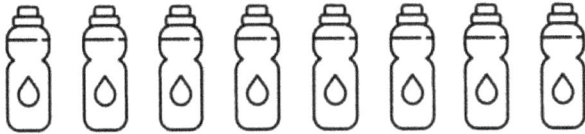

good *fine* *so/so* *bad* *horrible*
☐   ☐   ☐   ☐   ☐

water intake tracker

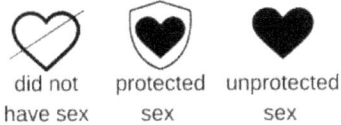

thoughts about how i'm feeling :

_____
_____
_____
_____

exercise

prenatal vitamin ☐

meals for the day

*breakfast*_____

*lunch*_____

*dinner*_____

*snacks*_____

Intercourse

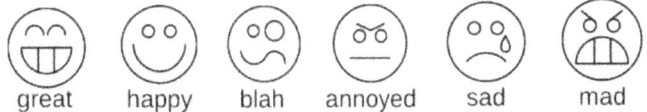

did not   protected   unprotected
have sex   sex   sex

Mood

great   happy   blah   annoyed   sad   mad

Symptoms

tender breasts   headache   backache   fatigue   cravings

cramps   acne   nausea   bloating   insomnia

constipation   diarrhea   joint pain   spotting   congestion

Date _____ # Daily Cycle Log Cycle Day_____

temperature _____ opk result _____ cervical fluid _____
(none, sticky, egg white, watery, unusual)

my mood today is...

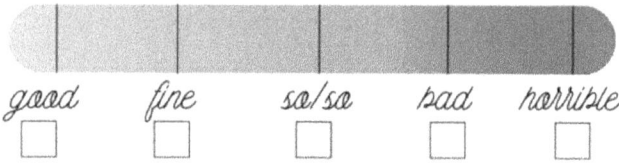

good   fine   so/so   bad   horrible
☐   ☐   ☐   ☐   ☐

water intake tracker

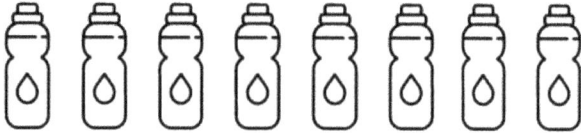

meals for the day

thoughts about how i'm feeling :

_____
_____
_____
_____

exercise

prenatal vitamin ⧉

breakfast_____

lunch_____

dinner_____

snacks_____

Intercourse

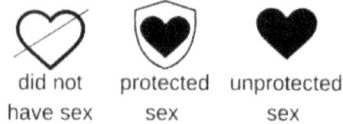

did not   protected   unprotected
have sex   sex   sex

Mood

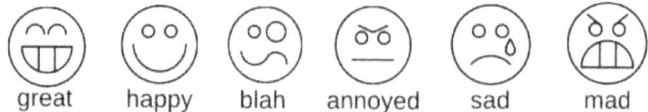

great   happy   blah   annoyed   sad   mad

Symptoms

tender breasts	headache	backache	fatigue	cravings
cramps	acne	nausea	bloating	insomnia
constipation	diarrhea	joint pain	spotting	congestion

Date _____ # Daily Cycle Log Cycle Day_____

temperature _____ opk result_____ cervical fluid _____
(none, sticky, egg white, watery, unusual)

my mood today is...

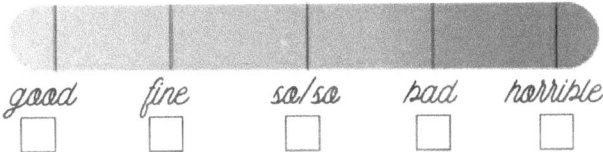

good   fine   so/so   bad   horrible
☐   ☐   ☐   ☐   ☐

thoughts about how i'm feeling :

_____
_____
_____
_____

water intake tracker

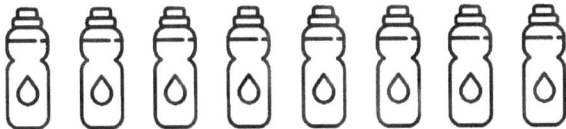

exercise
_____
| |
| |
| |
_____

meals for the day

prenatal vitamin ▢

breakfast_____
lunch_____
dinner_____
snacks_____

Intercourse

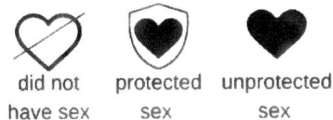

did not   protected   unprotected
have sex   sex   sex

Mood

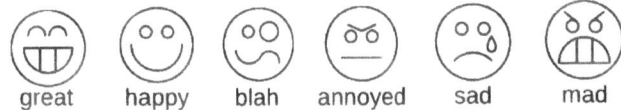

great   happy   blah   annoyed   sad   mad

Symptoms

tender breasts	headache	backache	fatigue	cravings
cramps	acne	nausea	bloating	insomnia
constipation	diarrhea	joint pain	spotting	congestion

Daily Cycle Log

Date _____   Cycle Day_____

temperature _____   opk result_____   cervical fluid _____
(none, sticky, egg white, watery, unusual)

my mood today is...

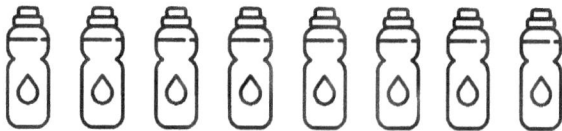

good   fine   so/so   bad   horrible
☐   ☐   ☐   ☐   ☐

water intake tracker

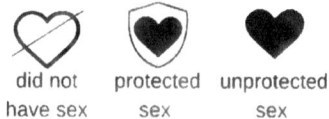

meals for the day

breakfast _____

lunch _____

dinner _____

snacks _____

thoughts about how i'm feeling :

_____

_____

_____

_____

exercise

prenatal vitamin ▢

Intercourse

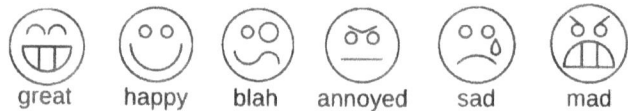

did not   protected   unprotected
have sex   sex   sex

Mood

great   happy   blah   annoyed   sad   mad

Symptoms

tender breasts	headache	backache	fatigue	cravings
cramps	acne	nausea	bloating	insomnia
constipation	diarrhea	joint pain	spotting	congestion

Date _____ # Daily Cycle Log Cycle Day_____

temperature _____   opk result_____   cervical fluid _____
(none, sticky, egg white, watery, unusual)

my mood today is...

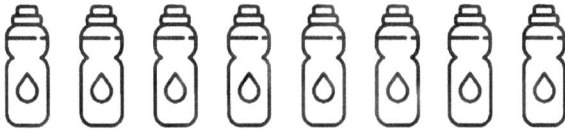

good *fine* *so/so* *bad* *horrible*
☐   ☐   ☐   ☐   ☐

water intake tracker

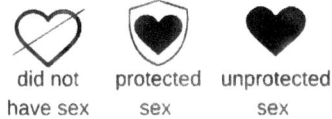

meals for the day

*breakfast*_____

*lunch*_____

*dinner*_____

*snacks*_____

thoughts about how i'm feeling :

_____

_____

_____

_____

exercise

prenatal vitamin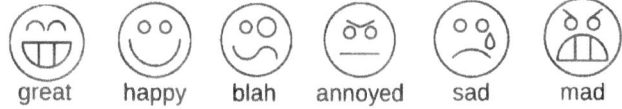

Intercourse

did not have sex   protected sex   unprotected sex

Mood

great   happy   blah   annoyed   sad   mad

Symptoms

tender breasts   headache   backache   fatigue   cravings

cramps   acne   nausea   bloating   insomnia

constipation   diarrhea   joint pain   spotting   congestion

Date _____ **Daily Cycle Log** Cycle Day_____

temperature _____ opk result _____ cervical fluid _____
(none, sticky, egg white, watery, unusual)

my mood today is...

good ☐   *fine* ☐   *so/so* ☐   *bad* ☐   *horrible* ☐

thoughts about how i'm feeling :

_____
_____
_____
_____

water intake tracker

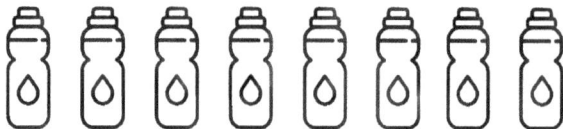

exercise

meals for the day

prenatal vitamin ▢

*breakfast*_____

*lunch*_____

*dinner*_____

*snacks*_____

Intercourse

did not have sex   protected sex   unprotected sex

Mood

great   happy   blah   annoyed   sad   mad

Symptoms

tender breasts	headache	backache	fatigue	cravings
cramps	acne	nausea	bloating	insomnia
constipation	diarrhea	joint pain	spotting	congestion

basal body temperature chart

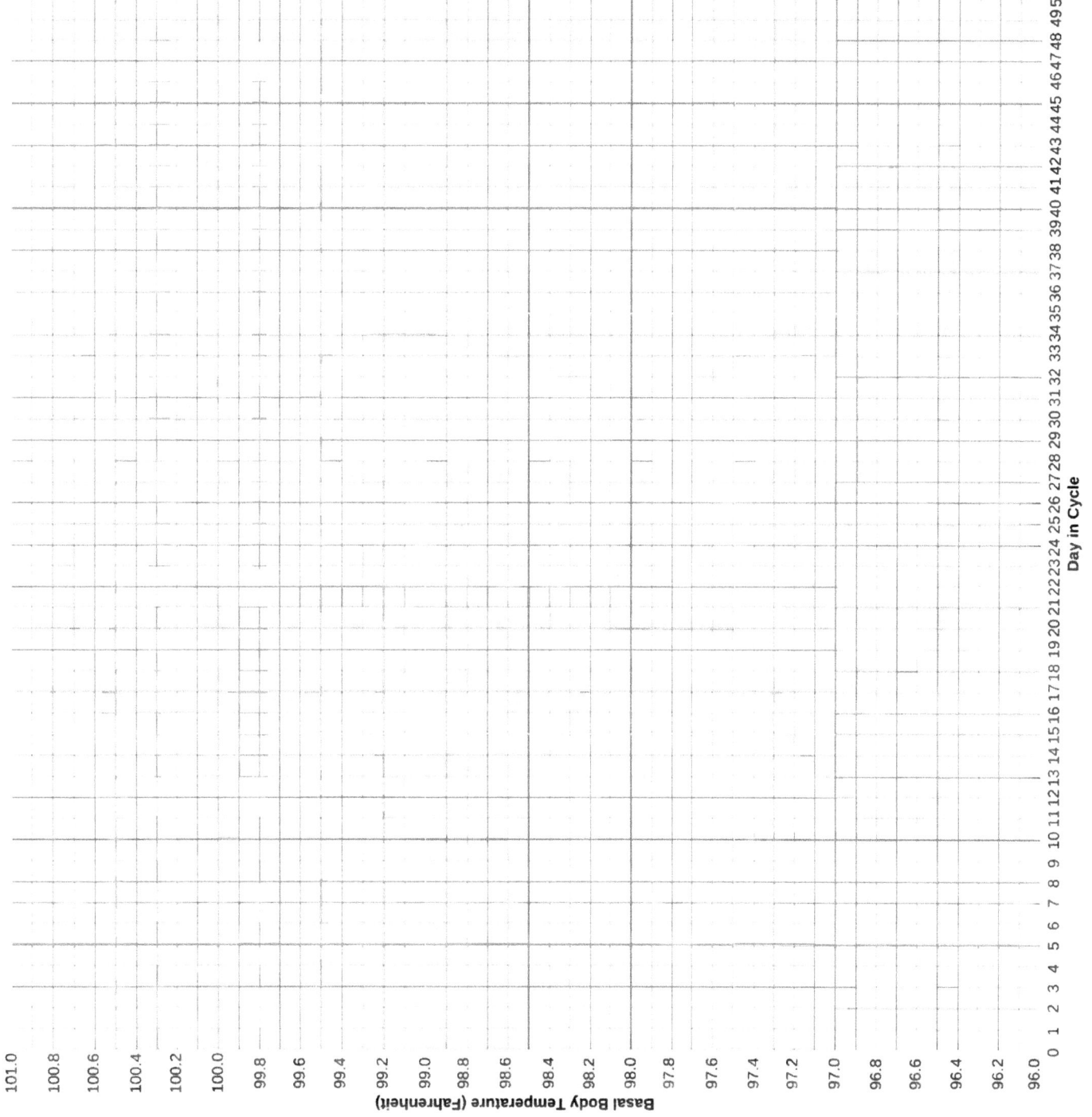

Basal Body Temperature (Fahrenheit)

101.0
100.8
100.6
100.4
100.2
100.0
99.8
99.6
99.4
99.2
99.0
98.8
98.6
98.4
98.2
98.0
97.8
97.6
97.4
97.2
97.0
96.8
96.6
96.4
96.2
96.0

0 1 2 3 4 5 6 7 8 9 10 11 12 13 14 15 16 17 18 19 20 21 22 23 24 25 26 27 28 29 30 31 32 33 34 35 36 37 38 39 40 41 42 43 44 45 46 47 48 49 50

Day in Cycle

Cycle tracker

first day of period _____

cycle number _____

August

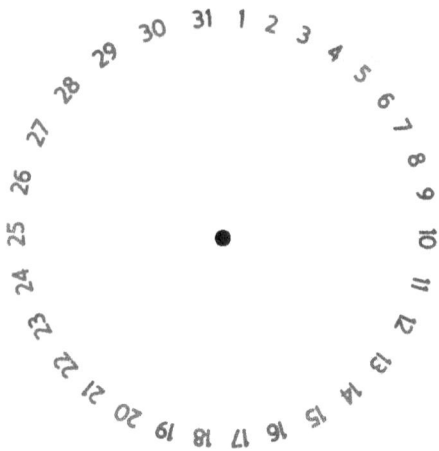

Menstruation Flow

Day 1	Day 2	Day 3
◊◊◊◊◊	◊◊◊◊◊	◊◊◊◊◊

Day 4	Day 5	Day 6
◊◊◊◊◊	◊◊◊◊◊	◊◊◊◊◊

Day 7

◊◊◊◊◊

Mood

Day 1	Day 2	Day 3	Day 4	Day 5	Day 6	Day 7
calm	calm	calm	calm	calm	calm	calm
happy	happy	happy	happy	happy	happy	happy
energetic	energetic	energetic	energetic	energetic	energetic	energetic
irritated	irritated	irritated	irritated	irritated	irritated	irritated
sad	sad	sad	sad	sad	sad	sad
anxious	anxious	anxious	anxious	anxious	anxious	anxious

Symptoms

Day 1	Day 2	Day 3	Day 4	Day 5	Day 6	Day 7
acne	acne	acne	acne	acne	acne	acne
nausea	nausea	nausea	nausea	nausea	nausea	nausea
cramps	cramps	cramps	cramps	cramps	cramps	cramps
headache	headache	headache	headache	headache	headache	headache
fatigue	fatigue	fatigue	fatigue	fatigue	fatigue	fatigue
bloating	bloating	bloating	bloating	bloating	bloating	bloating
back ache	back ache	back ache	back ache	back ache	back ache	back ache
sore boobs	sore boobs	sore boobs	sore boobs	sore boobs	sore boobs	sore boobs

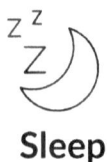

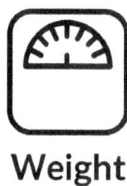

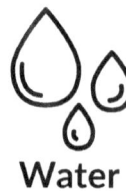

Sleep

_____

Weight

_____

Water

_____

1	
2	
3	
4	
5	
6	
7	
8	
9	
10	
11	
12	
13	
14	
15	
16	
17	
18	
19	
20	
21	
22	
23	
24	
25	
26	
27	
28	
29	
30	
31	

Notes:

Daily Cycle Log

Date _____   Cycle Day_____

temperature _____   opk result_____   cervical fluid _____
(none, sticky, egg white, watery, unusual)

my mood today is...

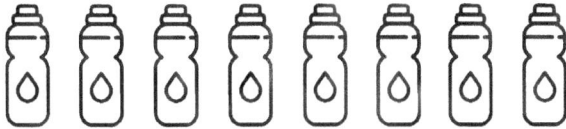

good	*fine*	*so/so*	*bad*	*horrible*
☐	☐	☐	☐	☐

thoughts about how i'm feeling :

_____

_____

_____

_____

water intake tracker

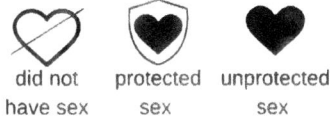

exercise

meals for the day

prenatal vitamin 🔲

*breakfast*_____

*lunch*_____

*dinner*_____

*snacks*_____

Intercourse

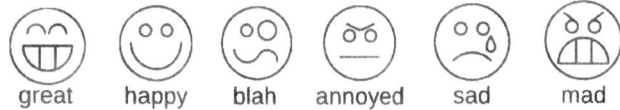

did not have sex   protected sex   unprotected sex

Mood

great   happy   blah   annoyed   sad   mad

Symptoms

tender breasts	headache	backache	fatigue	cravings
cramps	acne	nausea	bloating	insomnia
constipation	diarrhea	joint pain	spotting	congestion

Daily Cycle Log

Date _____   Cycle Day _____

temperature _____   opk result _____   cervical fluid _____
(none, sticky, egg white, watery, unusual)

my mood today is...

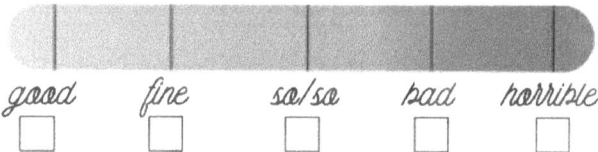

good   fine   so/so   bad   horrible
☐   ☐   ☐   ☐   ☐

thoughts about how i'm feeling :

_____

_____

_____

_____

exercise

water intake tracker

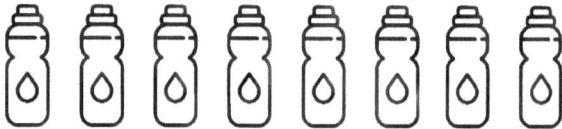

prenatal vitamin ▢

meals for the day

breakfast _____

lunch _____

dinner _____

snacks _____

Intercourse

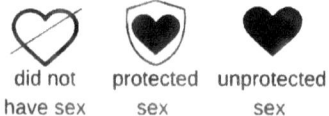

did not have sex   protected sex   unprotected sex

Mood

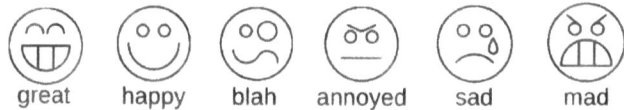

great   happy   blah   annoyed   sad   mad

Symptoms

tender breasts	headache	backache	fatigue	cravings
cramps	acne	nausea	bloating	insomnia
constipation	diarrhea	joint pain	spotting	congestion

Date _____ # Daily Cycle Log Cycle Day_____

temperature _____   opk result _____   cervical fluid _____
(none, sticky, egg white, watery, unusual)

my mood today is...

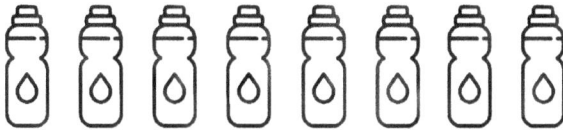

good   fine   so/so   bad   horrible
☐   ☐   ☐   ☐   ☐

water intake tracker

🍶 🍶 🍶 🍶 🍶 🍶 🍶 🍶

meals for the day

thoughts about how i'm feeling :

_____
_____
_____
_____

exercise

prenatal vitamin 🔲

breakfast _____
lunch _____
dinner _____
snacks _____

Intercourse   ## Mood

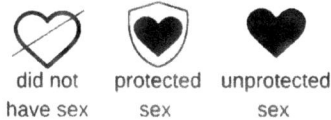

did not   protected   unprotected
have sex   sex   sex

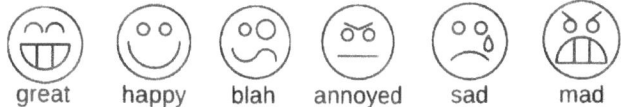

great   happy   blah   annoyed   sad   mad

Symptoms

tender breasts	headache	backache	fatigue	cravings
cramps	acne	nausea	bloating	insomnia
constipation	diarrhea	joint pain	spotting	congestion

Date _____ **Daily Cycle Log** Cycle Day_____

temperature _____   opk result _____   cervical fluid _____
(none, sticky, egg white, watery, unusual)

my mood today is...

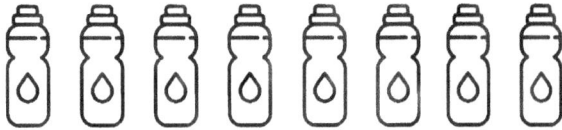

good *fine* *so/so* *bad* *horrible*
☐   ☐   ☐   ☐   ☐

water intake tracker

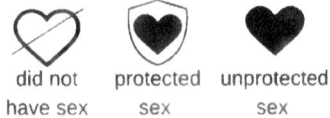

thoughts about how i'm feeling :

_____
_____
_____
_____

exercise

meals for the day

prenatal vitamin ⧉

*breakfast*_____

*lunch*_____

*dinner*_____

*snacks*_____

Intercourse

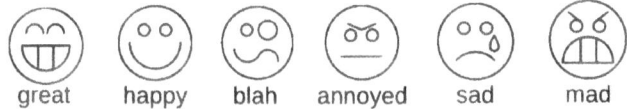

did not   protected   unprotected
have sex   sex   sex

Mood

😁   🙂   😛   😠   😢   😡
great   happy   blah   annoyed   sad   mad

Symptoms

tender breasts	headache	backache	fatigue	cravings
cramps	acne	nausea	bloating	insomnia
constipation	diarrhea	joint pain	spotting	congestion

Date _____ # Daily Cycle Log Cycle Day_____

temperature _____   opk result_____   cervical fluid _____
(none, sticky, egg white, watery, unusual)

my mood today is...

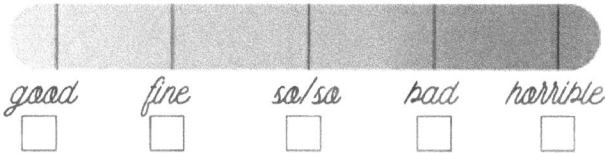

good   fine   so/so   bad   horrible
☐   ☐   ☐   ☐   ☐

water intake tracker

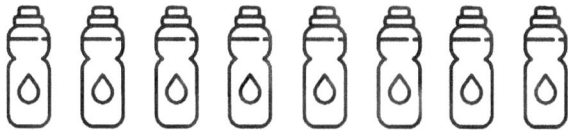

thoughts about how i'm feeling :

_____
_____
_____
_____

exercise

prenatal vitamin 🗆

meals for the day

breakfast_____

lunch_____

dinner_____

snacks_____

Intercourse

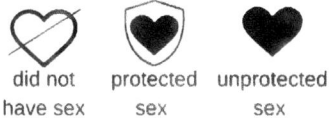

did not   protected   unprotected
have sex   sex   sex

Mood

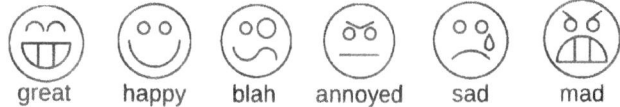

great   happy   blah   annoyed   sad   mad

Symptoms

tender breasts	headache	backache	fatigue	cravings
cramps	acne	nausea	bloating	insomnia
constipation	diarrhea	joint pain	spotting	congestion

Date _____ # Daily Cycle Log Cycle Day_____

temperature _____   opk result _____   cervical fluid _____
(none, sticky, egg white, watery, unusual)

my mood today is...

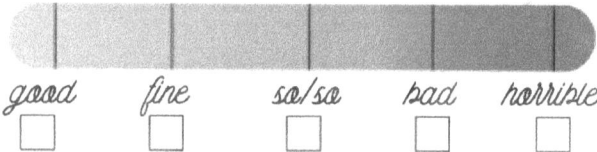

good fine so/so bad horrible
☐   ☐   ☐   ☐   ☐

thoughts about how i'm feeling :

_____

_____

_____

_____

water intake tracker

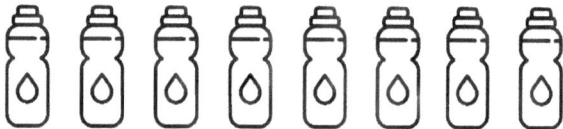

exercise

meals for the day

prenatal vitamin 🗋

breakfast _____

lunch _____

dinner _____

snacks _____

Intercourse

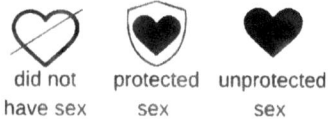

did not have sex   protected sex   unprotected sex

Mood

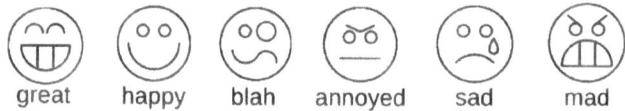

great   happy   blah   annoyed   sad   mad

Symptoms

tender breasts	headache	backache	fatigue	cravings
cramps	acne	nausea	bloating	insomnia
constipation	diarrhea	joint pain	spotting	congestion

Date _____ # Daily Cycle Log Cycle Day_____

temperature _____   opk result _____   cervical fluid _____

(none, sticky, egg white, watery, unusual)

my mood today is...

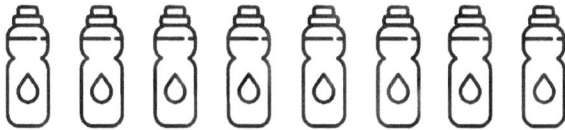

good ☐   *fine* ☐   *so/so* ☐   *bad* ☐   *horrible* ☐

thoughts about how i'm feeling :

_____

_____

_____

_____

water intake tracker

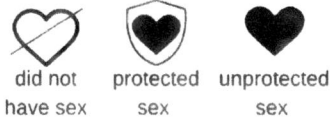

exercise
```
┌─────────────────────────────┐
│                             │
│                             │
│                             │
└─────────────────────────────┘
```

meals for the day

prenatal vitamin 📑

breakfast _____

lunch _____

dinner _____

snacks _____

Intercourse

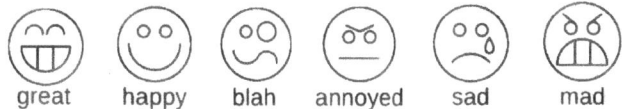

did not have sex   protected sex   unprotected sex

Mood

great   happy   blah   annoyed   sad   mad

Symptoms

tender breasts	headache	backache	fatigue	cravings
cramps	acne	nausea	bloating	insomnia
constipation	diarrhea	joint pain	spotting	congestion

date range _____

cycle # _____

basal body temperature chart

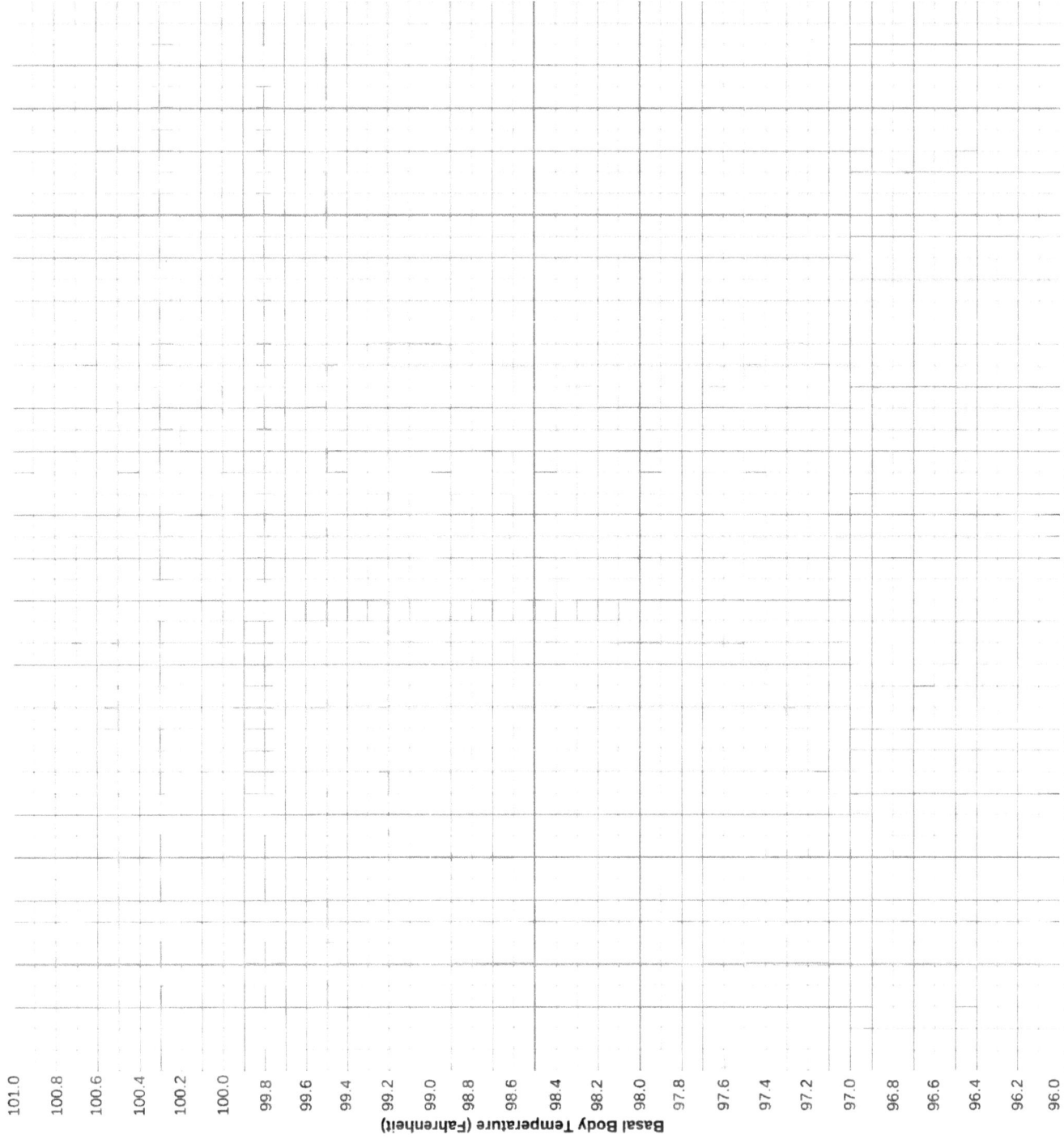

Basal Body Temperature (Fahrenheit)

| 101.0 |
| 100.8 |
| 100.6 |
| 100.4 |
| 100.2 |
| 100.0 |
| 99.8 |
| 99.6 |
| 99.4 |
| 99.2 |
| 99.0 |
| 98.8 |
| 98.6 |
| 98.4 |
| 98.2 |
| 98.0 |
| 97.8 |
| 97.6 |
| 97.4 |
| 97.2 |
| 97.0 |
| 96.8 |
| 96.6 |
| 96.4 |
| 96.2 |
| 96.0 |

0 1 2 3 4 5 6 7 8 9 10 11 12 13 14 15 16 17 18 19 20 21 22 23 24 25 26 27 28 29 30 31 32 33 34 35 36 37 38 39 40 41 42 43 44 45 46 47 48 49 50

Day in Cycle

Cycle tracker

first day of period _____

cycle number _____

September

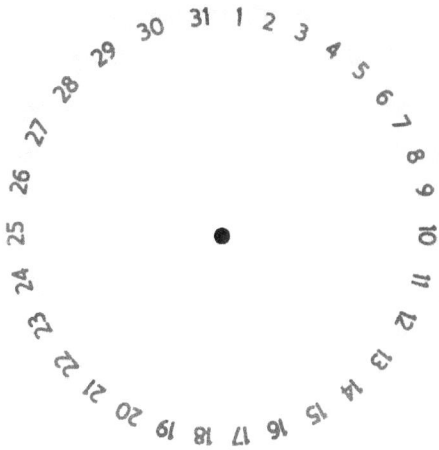

Menstruation Flow

Day 1	Day 2	Day 3
⬠⬠⬠⬠⬠	⬠⬠⬠⬠⬠	⬠⬠⬠⬠⬠

Day 4	Day 5	Day 6
⬠⬠⬠⬠⬠	⬠⬠⬠⬠⬠	⬠⬠⬠⬠⬠

Day 7

⬠⬠⬠⬠⬠

Mood

Day 1	Day 2	Day 3	Day 4	Day 5	Day 6	Day 7
calm	calm	calm	calm	calm	calm	calm
happy	happy	happy	happy	happy	happy	happy
energetic	energetic	energetic	energetic	energetic	energetic	energetic
irritated	irritated	irritated	irritated	irritated	irritated	irritated
sad	sad	sad	sad	sad	sad	sad
anxious	anxious	anxious	anxious	anxious	anxious	anxious

Symptoms

Day 1	Day 2	Day 3	Day 4	Day 5	Day 6	Day 7
acne	acne	acne	acne	acne	acne	acne
nausea	nausea	nausea	nausea	nausea	nausea	nausea
cramps	cramps	cramps	cramps	cramps	cramps	cramps
headache	headache	headache	headache	headache	headache	headache
fatigue	fatigue	fatigue	fatigue	fatigue	fatigue	fatigue
bloating	bloating	bloating	bloating	bloating	bloating	bloating
back ache	back ache	back ache	back ache	back ache	back ache	back ache
sore boobs	sore boobs	sore boobs	sore boobs	sore boobs	sore boobs	sore boobs

Sleep

Weight

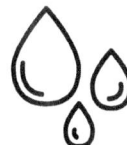

Water

1	
2	
3	
4	
5	
6	
7	
8	
9	
10	
11	
12	
13	
14	
15	
16	
17	
18	
19	
20	
21	
22	
23	
24	
25	
26	
27	
28	
29	
30	
31	

Notes:

Date _____   # Daily Cycle Log   Cycle Day_____

temperature _____   opk result _____   cervical fluid _____
(none, sticky, egg white, watery, unusual)

my mood today is...

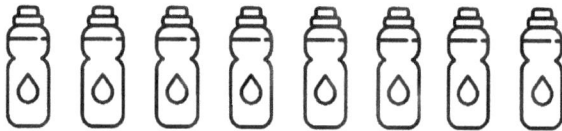

good   fine   so/so   bad   horrible
☐   ☐   ☐   ☐   ☐

thoughts about how i'm feeling :

_____
_____
_____
_____

exercise

water intake tracker

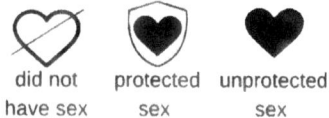

meals for the day

prenatal vitamin ▢

breakfast _____

lunch _____

dinner _____

snacks _____

Intercourse

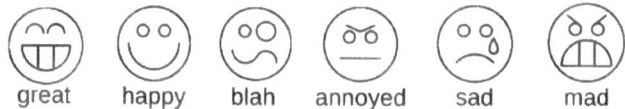

did not   protected   unprotected
have sex   sex   sex

Mood

great   happy   blah   annoyed   sad   mad

Symptoms

tender breasts   headache   backache   fatigue   cravings

cramps   acne   nausea   bloating   insomnia

constipation   diarrhea   joint pain   spotting   congestion

Daily Cycle Log

Date _____

Cycle Day _____

temperature _____   opk result _____   cervical fluid _____
(none, sticky, egg white, watery, unusual)

my mood today is...

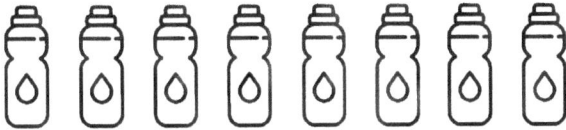

good   fine   so/so   bad   horrible
☐   ☐   ☐   ☐   ☐

thoughts about how i'm feeling :

_____

_____

_____

_____

water intake tracker

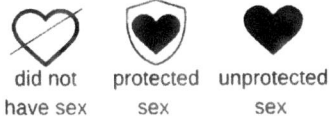

exercise
_____

meals for the day

prenatal vitamin 🗌

breakfast _____

lunch _____

dinner _____

snacks _____

Intercourse

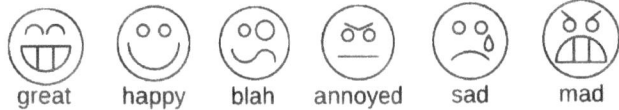

did not have sex   protected sex   unprotected sex

Mood

great   happy   blah   annoyed   sad   mad

Symptoms

tender breasts	headache	backache	fatigue	cravings
cramps	acne	nausea	bloating	insomnia
constipation	diarrhea	joint pain	spotting	congestion

Daily Cycle Log

Date _____   Cycle Day _____

temperature _____   opk result _____   cervical fluid _____
(none, sticky, egg white, watery, unusual)

my mood today is...

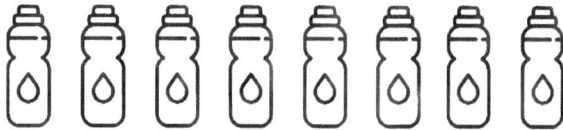

good   *fine*   *so/so*   *bad*   *horrible*
☐   ☐   ☐   ☐   ☐

thoughts about how i'm feeling :

_____

_____

_____

_____

water intake tracker

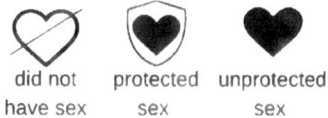

exercise

meals for the day

prenatal vitamin ☐

breakfast _____

lunch _____

dinner _____

snacks _____

Intercourse

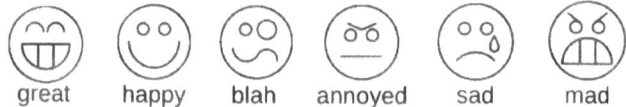

did not have sex   protected sex   unprotected sex

Mood

great   happy   blah   annoyed   sad   mad

Symptoms

tender breasts	headache	backache	fatigue	cravings
cramps	acne	nausea	bloating	insomnia
constipation	diarrhea	joint pain	spotting	congestion

Daily Cycle Log

Date _____   Cycle Day _____

temperature _____   opk result _____   cervical fluid _____
(none, sticky, egg white, watery, unusual)

my mood today is...

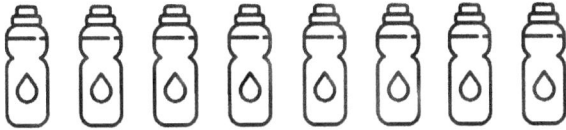

good   fine   so/so   bad   horrible
☐   ☐   ☐   ☐   ☐

water intake tracker

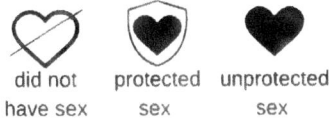

thoughts about how i'm feeling :

_____

_____

_____

_____

exercise

prenatal vitamin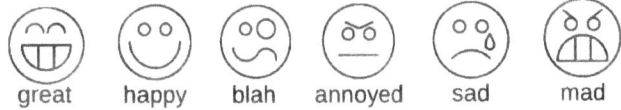

meals for the day

breakfast _____

lunch _____

dinner _____

snacks _____

Intercourse

did not   protected   unprotected
have sex   sex   sex

Mood

great   happy   blah   annoyed   sad   mad

Symptoms

tender breasts	headache	backache	fatigue	cravings
cramps	acne	nausea	bloating	insomnia
constipation	diarrhea	joint pain	spotting	congestion

Daily Cycle Log

Date _____   Cycle Day_____

temperature _____   opk result _____   cervical fluid _____
(none, sticky, egg white, watery, unusual)

my mood today is...

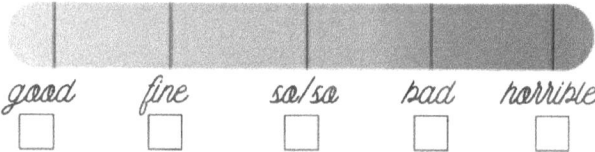

good ☐   fine ☐   so/so ☐   bad ☐   horrible ☐

water intake tracker

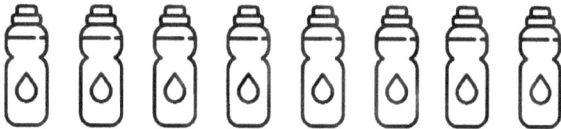

thoughts about how i'm feeling :

_____

_____

_____

_____

exercise

prenatal vitamin

meals for the day

breakfast _____

lunch _____

dinner _____

snacks _____

Intercourse

did not have sex   protected sex   unprotected sex

Mood

great   happy   blah   annoyed   sad   mad

Symptoms

tender breasts	headache	backache	fatigue	cravings
cramps	acne	nausea	bloating	insomnia
constipation	diarrhea	joint pain	spotting	congestion

Date _____ # Daily Cycle Log Cycle Day _____

temperature _____ opk result _____ cervical fluid _____
(none, sticky, egg white, watery, unusual)

my mood today is...

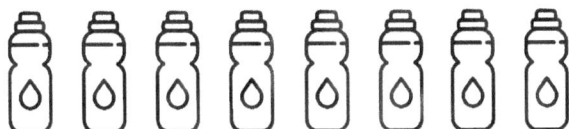

good *fine* *so/so* *bad* *horrible*
☐ ☐ ☐ ☐ ☐

thoughts about how i'm feeling :

_____
_____
_____
_____

water intake tracker

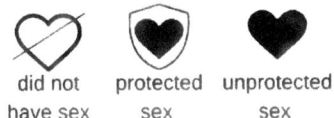

exercise

meals for the day

prenatal vitamin ▢

breakfast _____

lunch _____

dinner _____

snacks _____

Intercourse

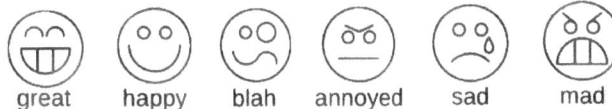

did not have sex | protected sex | unprotected sex

Mood

great happy blah annoyed sad mad

Symptoms

tender breasts	headache	backache	fatigue	cravings
cramps	acne	nausea	bloating	insomnia
constipation	diarrhea	joint pain	spotting	congestion

Daily Cycle Log

Date _____   Cycle Day _____

temperature _____   opk result _____   cervical fluid _____
(none, sticky, egg white, watery, unusual)

my mood today is...

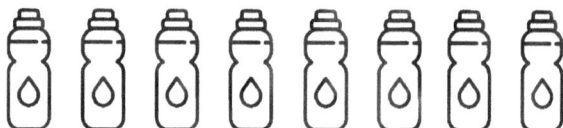

good ☐   fine ☐   so/so ☐   bad ☐   horrible ☐

thoughts about how i'm feeling :

_____
_____
_____
_____

water intake tracker

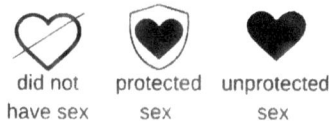

exercise
_____

meals for the day

prenatal vitamin 🗒

breakfast _____

lunch _____

dinner _____

snacks _____

Intercourse

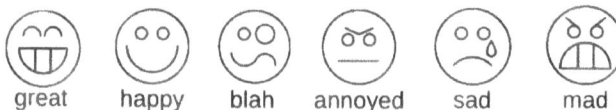

did not have sex   protected sex   unprotected sex

Mood

great   happy   blah   annoyed   sad   mad

Symptoms

tender breasts	headache	backache	fatigue	cravings
cramps	acne	nausea	bloating	insomnia
constipation	diarrhea	joint pain	spotting	congestion

date range _____

basal body temperature chart

cycle # _____

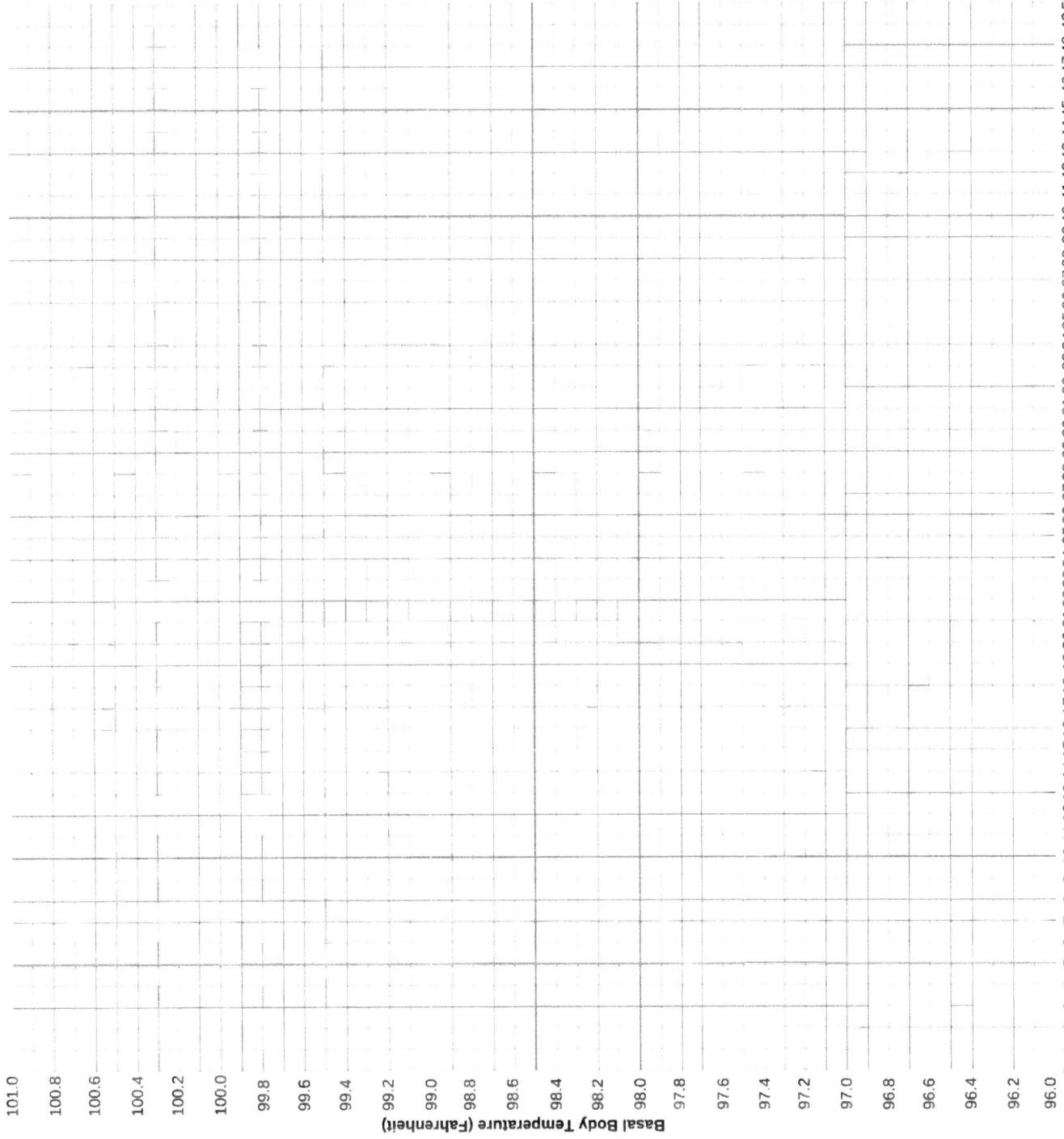

Basal Body Temperature (Fahrenheit)

| 101.0 |
| 100.8 |
| 100.6 |
| 100.4 |
| 100.2 |
| 100.0 |
| 99.8 |
| 99.6 |
| 99.4 |
| 99.2 |
| 99.0 |
| 98.8 |
| 98.6 |
| 98.4 |
| 98.2 |
| 98.0 |
| 97.8 |
| 97.6 |
| 97.4 |
| 97.2 |
| 97.0 |
| 96.8 |
| 96.6 |
| 96.4 |
| 96.2 |
| 96.0 |

0 1 2 3 4 5 6 7 8 9 10 11 12 13 14 15 16 17 18 19 20 21 22 23 24 25 26 27 28 29 30 31 32 33 34 35 36 37 38 39 40 41 42 43 44 45 46 47 48 49 50

Day in Cycle

Cycle tracker

first day of period _____

cycle number _____

October

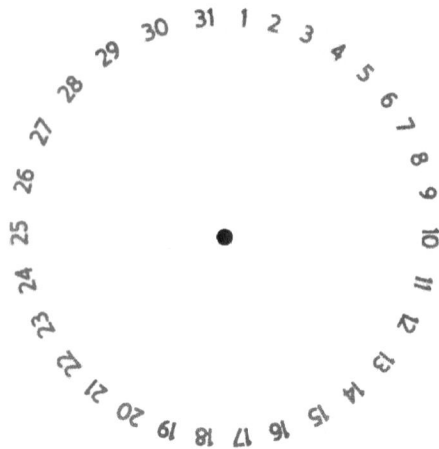

Menstruation Flow

Day 1	Day 2	Day 3
◊◊◊◊◊	◊◊◊◊◊	◊◊◊◊◊

Day 4	Day 5	Day 6
◊◊◊◊◊	◊◊◊◊◊	◊◊◊◊◊

Day 7
◊◊◊◊◊

Mood

Day 1	Day 2	Day 3	Day 4	Day 5	Day 6	Day 7
calm	calm	calm	calm	calm	calm	calm
happy	happy	happy	happy	happy	happy	happy
energetic	energetic	energetic	energetic	energetic	energetic	energetic
irritated	irritated	irritated	irritated	irritated	irritated	irritated
sad	sad	sad	sad	sad	sad	sad
anxious	anxious	anxious	anxious	anxious	anxious	anxious

Symptoms

Day 1	Day 2	Day 3	Day 4	Day 5	Day 6	Day 7
acne	acne	acne	acne	acne	acne	acne
nausea	nausea	nausea	nausea	nausea	nausea	nausea
cramps	cramps	cramps	cramps	cramps	cramps	cramps
headache	headache	headache	headache	headache	headache	headache
fatigue	fatigue	fatigue	fatigue	fatigue	fatigue	fatigue
bloating	bloating	bloating	bloating	bloating	bloating	bloating
back ache	back ache	back ache	back ache	back ache	back ache	back ache
sore boobs	sore boobs	sore boobs	sore boobs	sore boobs	sore boobs	sore boobs

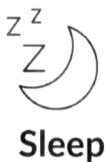

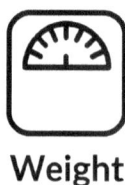

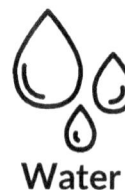

Sleep

Weight

Water

_____   _____   _____

1
2
3
4
5
6
7
8
9
10
11
12
13
14
15
16
17
18
19
20
21
22
23
24
25
26
27
28
29
30
31

Notes:

Date _____ **Daily Cycle Log** Cycle Day_____

temperature _____   opk result _____   cervical fluid _____
(none, sticky, egg white, watery, unusual)

my mood today is...

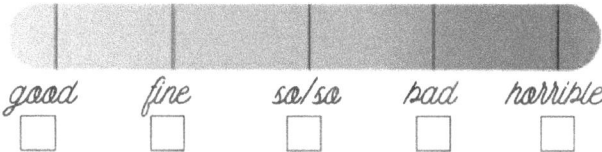

good   fine   so/so   bad   horrible
☐   ☐   ☐   ☐   ☐

thoughts about how i'm feeling :

_____

_____

_____

_____

water intake tracker

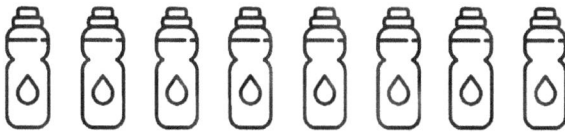

| exercise |
| |
| |
| |

meals for the day

prenatal vitamin 🗐

breakfast _____

lunch _____

dinner _____

snacks _____

Intercourse

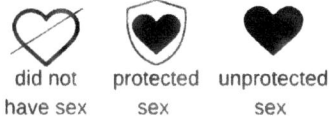

did not   protected   unprotected
have sex   sex   sex

Mood

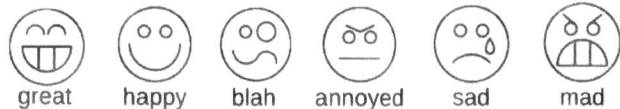

great   happy   blah   annoyed   sad   mad

Symptoms

tender breasts	headache	backache	fatigue	cravings
cramps	acne	nausea	bloating	insomnia
constipation	diarrhea	joint pain	spotting	congestion

Date _____   # Daily Cycle Log   Cycle Day _____

temperature _____   opk result _____   cervical fluid _____
(none, sticky, egg white, watery, unusual)

my mood today is...

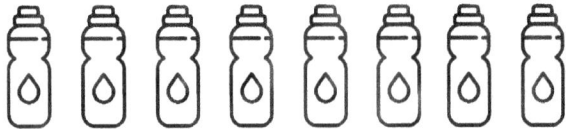

good   fine   so/so   bad   horrible
☐   ☐   ☐   ☐   ☐

water intake tracker

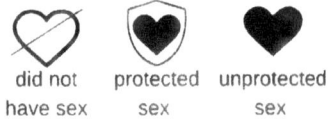

thoughts about how i'm feeling :

_____

_____

_____

_____

exercise

meals for the day

prenatal vitamin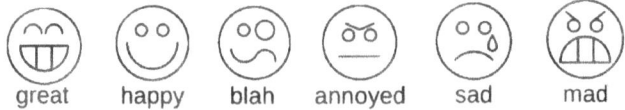

breakfast _____

lunch _____

dinner _____

snacks _____

Intercourse

did not have sex   protected sex   unprotected sex

Mood

great   happy   blah   annoyed   sad   mad

Symptoms

tender breasts   headache   backache   fatigue   cravings

cramps   acne   nausea   bloating   insomnia

constipation   diarrhea   joint pain   spotting   congestion

Date_____ # Daily Cycle Log Cycle Day_____

temperature _____   opk result_____   cervical fluid _____
(none, sticky, egg white, watery, unusual)

my mood today is...

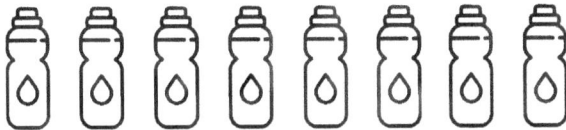

good   fine   so/so   bad   horrible
☐   ☐   ☐   ☐   ☐

water intake tracker

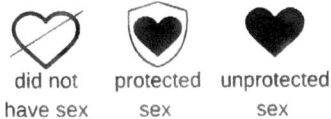

meals for the day

thoughts about how i'm feeling :

_____
_____
_____
_____

exercise

prenatal vitamin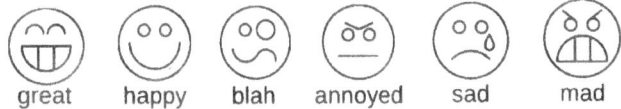

breakfast_____

lunch_____

dinner_____

snacks_____

Intercourse

did not   protected   unprotected
have sex   sex   sex

Mood

great   happy   blah   annoyed   sad   mad

Symptoms

tender breasts	headache	backache	fatigue	cravings
cramps	acne	nausea	bloating	insomnia
constipation	diarrhea	joint pain	spotting	congestion

Daily Cycle Log

Date _____   Cycle Day _____

temperature _____   opk result _____   cervical fluid _____
(none, sticky, egg white, watery, unusual)

my mood today is...

good ☐   fine ☐   so/so ☐   bad ☐   horrible ☐

water intake tracker

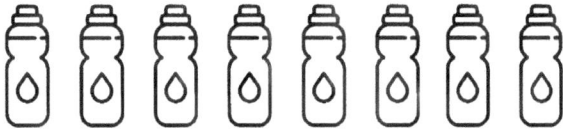

thoughts about how i'm feeling :

_____

_____

_____

_____

exercise

prenatal vitamin ❏

meals for the day

breakfast _____

lunch _____

dinner _____

snacks _____

Intercourse

did not have sex   protected sex   unprotected sex

Mood

great   happy   blah   annoyed   sad   mad

Symptoms

tender breasts	headache	backache	fatigue	cravings
cramps	acne	nausea	bloating	insomnia
constipation	diarrhea	joint pain	spotting	congestion

Daily Cycle Log

Date _____

Cycle Day_____

temperature _____   opk result_____   cervical fluid _____
(none, sticky, egg white, watery, unusual)

my mood today is...

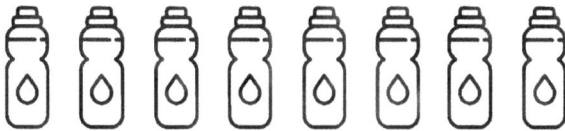

good ☐   *fine* ☐   *so/so* ☐   *bad* ☐   *horrible* ☐

thoughts about how i'm feeling :

_____

_____

_____

_____

water intake tracker

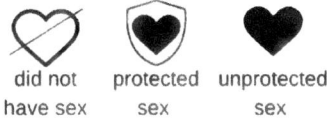

exercise

meals for the day

prenatal vitamin 🗐

*breakfast*_____

*lunch*_____

*dinner*_____

*snacks*_____

Intercourse

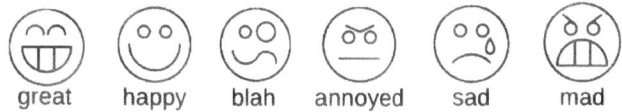

did not have sex   protected sex   unprotected sex

Mood

great   happy   blah   annoyed   sad   mad

Symptoms

tender breasts	headache	backache	fatigue	cravings
cramps	acne	nausea	bloating	insomnia
constipation	diarrhea	joint pain	spotting	congestion

Date _____ # Daily Cycle Log Cycle Day_____

temperature _____   opk result_____   cervical fluid _____
(none, sticky, egg white, watery, unusual)

my mood today is...

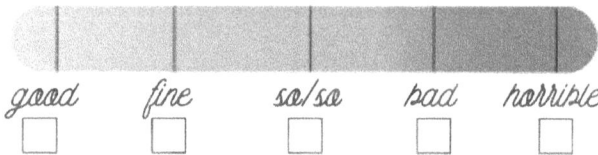

good   *fine*   *so/so*   *bad*   *horrible*
☐   ☐   ☐   ☐   ☐

thoughts about how i'm feeling :

_____
_____
_____
_____

water intake tracker

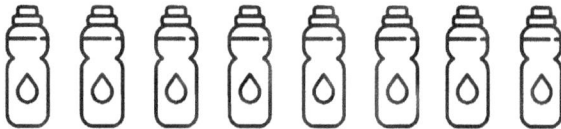

exercise

meals for the day   prenatal vitamin 🔲

*breakfast*_____

*lunch*_____

*dinner*_____

*snacks*_____

Intercourse

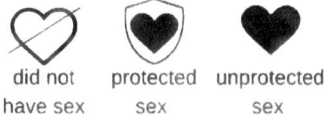

did not have sex   protected sex   unprotected sex

Mood

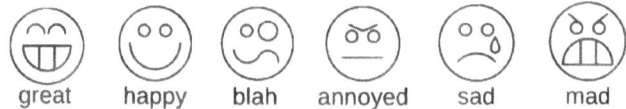

great   happy   blah   annoyed   sad   mad

Symptoms

tender breasts	headache	backache	fatigue	cravings
cramps	acne	nausea	bloating	insomnia
constipation	diarrhea	joint pain	spotting	congestion

Daily Cycle Log

Date _____   Cycle Day_____

temperature _____   opk result_____   cervical fluid _____
(none, sticky, egg white, watery, unusual)

my mood today is...

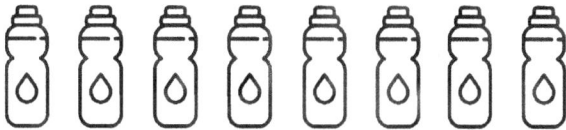

good   fine   so/so   bad   horrible
☐   ☐   ☐   ☐   ☐

thoughts about how i'm feeling :

_____

_____

_____

_____

water intake tracker

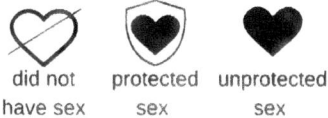

┌─────────────────────────────────────┐
│ exercise   │
│   │
│   │
│   │
└─────────────────────────────────────┘

meals for the day

prenatal vitamin ▱

breakfast_____

lunch_____

dinner_____

snacks_____

Intercourse

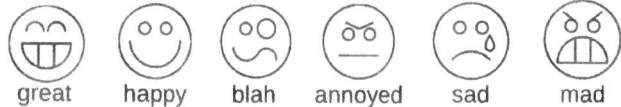

did not   protected   unprotected
have sex   sex   sex

Mood

great   happy   blah   annoyed   sad   mad

Symptoms

tender breasts	headache	backache	fatigue	cravings
cramps	acne	nausea	bloating	insomnia
constipation	diarrhea	joint pain	spotting	congestion

basal body temperature chart

Basal Body Temperature (Fahrenheit)

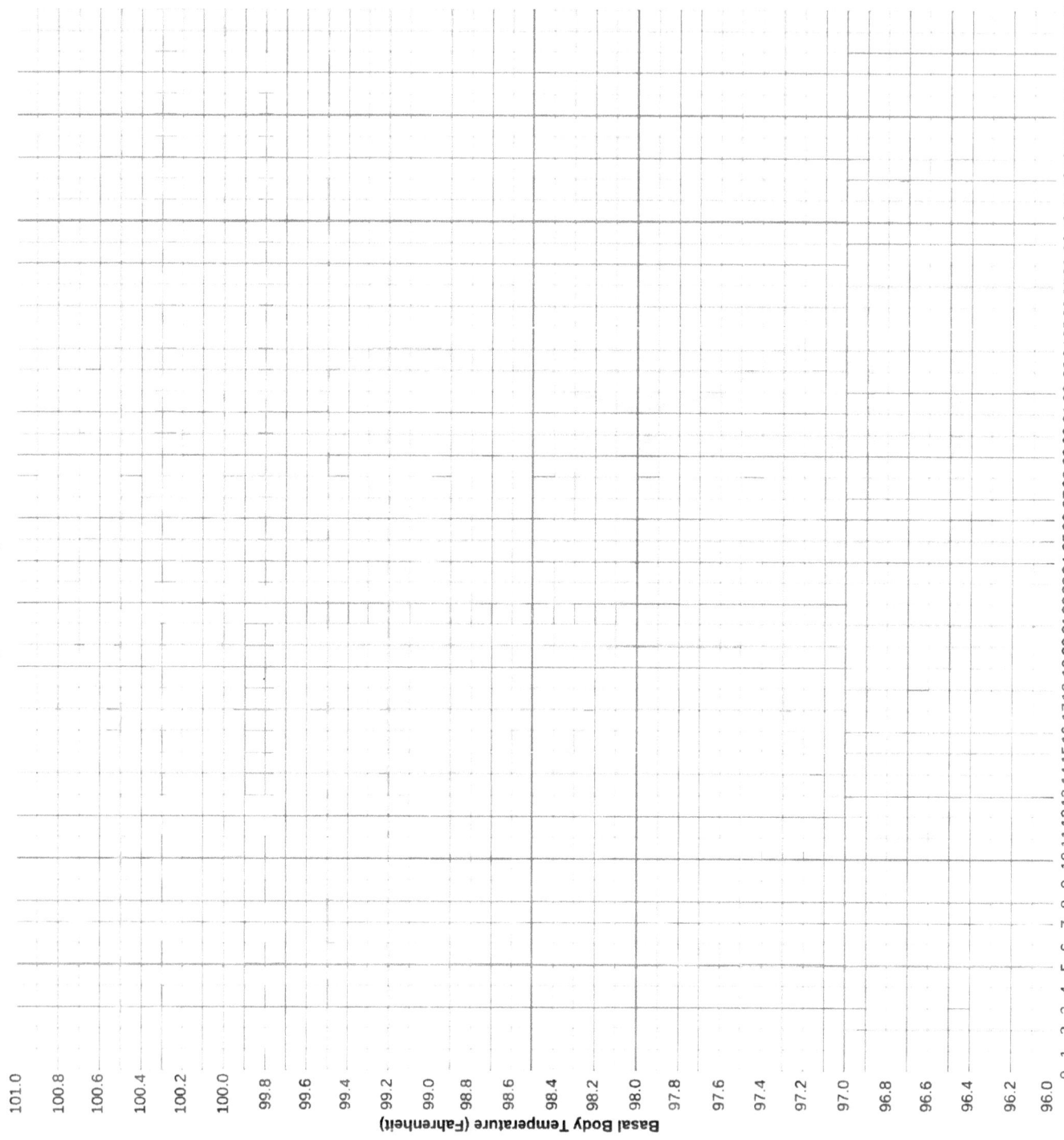

101.0
100.8
100.6
100.4
100.2
100.0
99.8
99.6
99.4
99.2
99.0
98.8
98.6
98.4
98.2
98.0
97.8
97.6
97.4
97.2
97.0
96.8
96.6
96.4
96.2
96.0

0 1 2 3 4 5 6 7 8 9 10 11 12 13 14 15 16 17 18 19 20 21 22 23 24 25 26 27 28 29 30 31 32 33 34 35 36 37 38 39 40 41 42 43 44 45 46 47 48 49 50

Day in Cycle

Cycle tracker

first day of period _____

cycle number _____

November

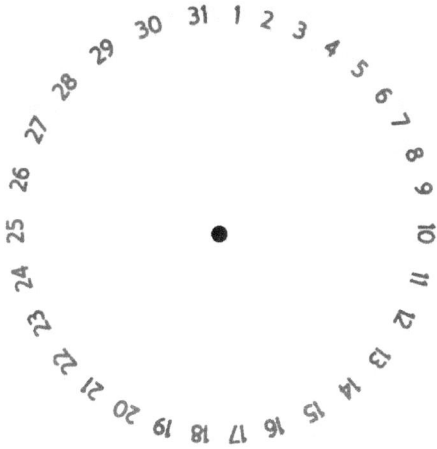

Menstruation Flow

Day 1	Day 2	Day 3
◇◇◇◇◇	◇◇◇◇◇	◇◇◇◇◇

Day 4	Day 5	Day 6
◇◇◇◇◇	◇◇◇◇◇	◇◇◇◇◇

Day 7
◇◇◇◇◇

Mood

Day 1	Day 2	Day 3	Day 4	Day 5	Day 6	Day 7
calm	calm	calm	calm	calm	calm	calm
happy	happy	happy	happy	happy	happy	happy
energetic	energetic	energetic	energetic	energetic	energetic	energetic
irritated	irritated	irritated	irritated	irritated	irritated	irritated
sad	sad	sad	sad	sad	sad	sad
anxious	anxious	anxious	anxious	anxious	anxious	anxious

Symptoms

Day 1	Day 2	Day 3	Day 4	Day 5	Day 6	Day 7
acne	acne	acne	acne	acne	acne	acne
nausea	nausea	nausea	nausea	nausea	nausea	nausea
cramps	cramps	cramps	cramps	cramps	cramps	cramps
headache	headache	headache	headache	headache	headache	headache
fatigue	fatigue	fatigue	fatigue	fatigue	fatigue	fatigue
bloating	bloating	bloating	bloating	bloating	bloating	bloating
back ache	back ache	back ache	back ache	back ache	back ache	back ache
sore boobs	sore boobs	sore boobs	sore boobs	sore boobs	sore boobs	sore boobs

1
2
3
4
5
6
7
8
9
10
11
12
13
14
15
16
17
18
19
20
21
22
23
24
25
26
27
28
29
30
31

Notes:

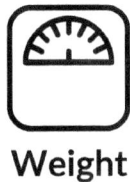

Sleep

_____

Weight

_____

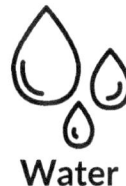

Water

_____

Date _____   # Daily Cycle Log   Cycle Day _____

temperature _____   opk result _____   cervical fluid _____
(none, sticky, egg white, watery, unusual)

my mood today is...

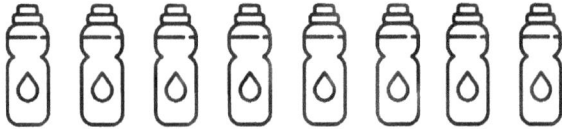

good   fine   so/so   bad   horrible
☐   ☐   ☐   ☐   ☐

thoughts about how i'm feeling :

_____

_____

_____

_____

water intake tracker

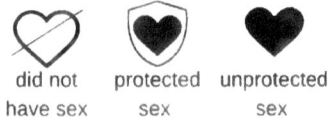

┌─────────────────────────────────────┐
│ exercise   │
│   │
│   │
└─────────────────────────────────────┘

meals for the day

prenatal vitamin 🗔

breakfast _____

lunch _____

dinner _____

snacks _____

Intercourse

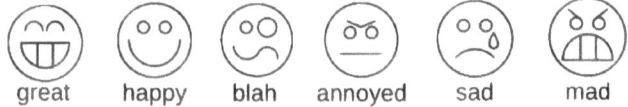

did not have sex   protected sex   unprotected sex

Mood

great   happy   blah   annoyed   sad   mad

Symptoms

tender breasts	headache	backache	fatigue	cravings
cramps	acne	nausea	bloating	insomnia
constipation	diarrhea	joint pain	spotting	congestion

Daily Cycle Log

Date _____ Cycle Day_____

temperature _____ opk result _____ cervical fluid _____
(none, sticky, egg white, watery, unusual)

my mood today is...

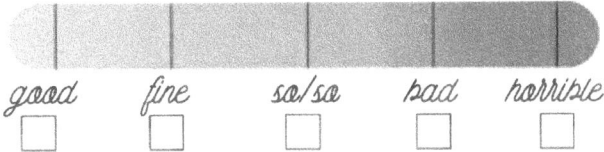

good   fine   so/so   bad   horrible
☐   ☐   ☐   ☐   ☐

thoughts about how i'm feeling :

_____
_____
_____
_____

water intake tracker

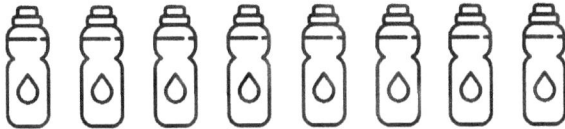

exercise

meals for the day

prenatal vitamin 🗐

breakfast _____
lunch _____
dinner _____
snacks _____

Intercourse

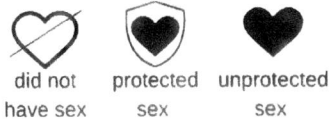

did not   protected   unprotected
have sex   sex   sex

Mood

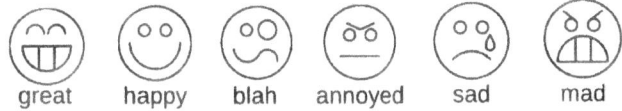

great   happy   blah   annoyed   sad   mad

Symptoms

tender breasts	headache	backache	fatigue	cravings
cramps	acne	nausea	bloating	insomnia
constipation	diarrhea	joint pain	spotting	congestion

Daily Cycle Log

Date _____   Cycle Day _____

temperature _____   opk result _____   cervical fluid _____
(none, sticky, egg white, watery, unusual)

my mood today is...

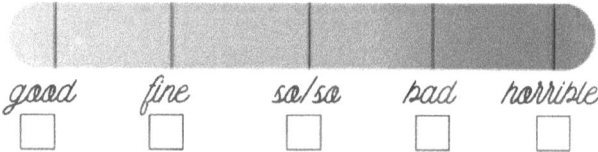

good *fine* *so/so* *bad* *horrible*
☐ ☐ ☐ ☐ ☐

water intake tracker

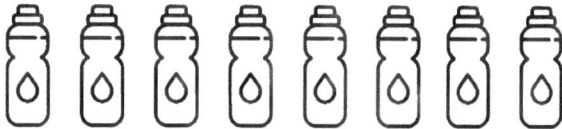

meals for the day

breakfast _____

lunch _____

dinner _____

snacks _____

thoughts about how i'm feeling :

_____

_____

_____

_____

exercise

prenatal vitamin ▢

Intercourse

did not have sex   protected sex   unprotected sex

Mood

great   happy   blah   annoyed   sad   mad

Symptoms

tender breasts	headache	backache	fatigue	cravings
cramps	acne	nausea	bloating	insomnia
constipation	diarrhea	joint pain	spotting	congestion

Daily Cycle Log

Date _____   Cycle Day_____

temperature _____   opk result_____   cervical fluid _____

(none, sticky, egg white, watery, unusual)

my mood today is...

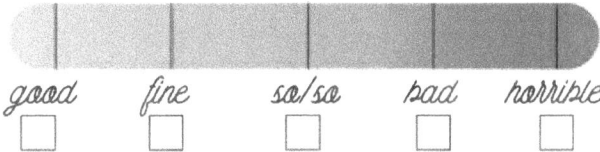

good   fine   so/so   bad   horrible
☐   ☐   ☐   ☐   ☐

thoughts about how i'm feeling :

_____
_____
_____
_____

water intake tracker

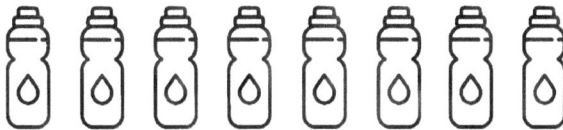

exercise

meals for the day

prenatal vitamin

breakfast _____

lunch _____

dinner _____

snacks _____

Intercourse

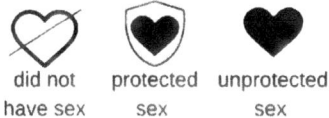

did not have sex   protected sex   unprotected sex

Mood

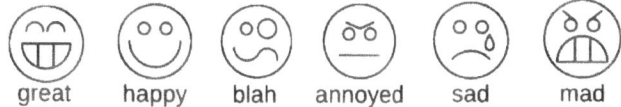

great   happy   blah   annoyed   sad   mad

Symptoms

tender breasts	headache	backache	fatigue	cravings
cramps	acne	nausea	bloating	insomnia
constipation	diarrhea	joint pain	spotting	congestion

Daily Cycle Log

Date _____   Cycle Day _____

temperature _____   opk result _____   cervical fluid _____
(none, sticky, egg white, watery, unusual)

my mood today is...

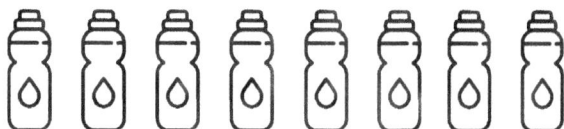

good ☐   fine ☐   so/so ☐   bad ☐   horrible ☐

thoughts about how i'm feeling :

_____

_____

_____

_____

water intake tracker

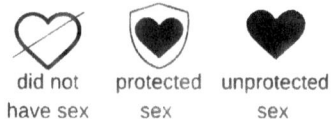

exercise

meals for the day

prenatal vitamin 🔲

breakfast _____

lunch _____

dinner _____

snacks _____

Intercourse

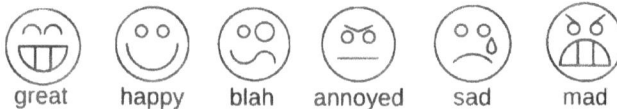

did not have sex   protected sex   unprotected sex

Mood

great   happy   blah   annoyed   sad   mad

Symptoms

tender breasts	headache	backache	fatigue	cravings
cramps	acne	nausea	bloating	insomnia
constipation	diarrhea	joint pain	spotting	congestion

Date _____   # Daily Cycle Log   Cycle Day _____

temperature _____   opk result _____   cervical fluid _____
(none, sticky, egg white, watery, unusual)

my mood today is...

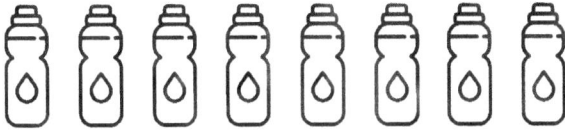

good   fine   so/so   bad   horrible
☐   ☐   ☐   ☐   ☐

thoughts about how i'm feeling :

_____

_____

_____

_____

water intake tracker

🍶 🍶 🍶 🍶 🍶 🍶 🍶 🍶

exercise
_____

meals for the day

prenatal vitamin ▢

breakfast _____

lunch _____

dinner _____

snacks _____

Intercourse

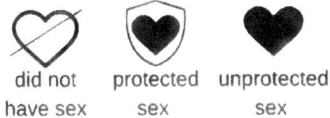

did not have sex   protected sex   unprotected sex

Mood

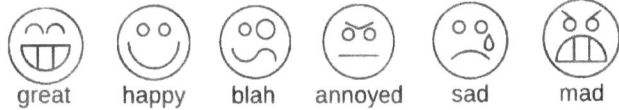

great   happy   blah   annoyed   sad   mad

Symptoms

tender breasts	headache	backache	fatigue	cravings
cramps	acne	nausea	bloating	insomnia
constipation	diarrhea	joint pain	spotting	congestion

Daily Cycle Log

Date _____   Cycle Day _____

temperature _____   opk result _____   cervical fluid _____
(none, sticky, egg white, watery, unusual)

my mood today is...

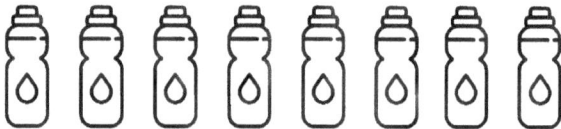

good ☐   fine ☐   so/so ☐   bad ☐   horrible ☐

thoughts about how i'm feeling :

_____
_____
_____
_____

water intake tracker

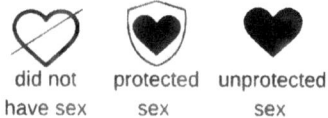

exercise
[ ]

meals for the day

prenatal vitamin ▢

breakfast _____
lunch _____
dinner _____
snacks _____

Intercourse

did not have sex   protected sex   unprotected sex

Mood

great   happy   blah   annoyed   sad   mad

Symptoms

tender breasts	headache	backache	fatigue	cravings
cramps	acne	nausea	bloating	insomnia
constipation	diarrhea	joint pain	spotting	congestion

basal body temperature chart

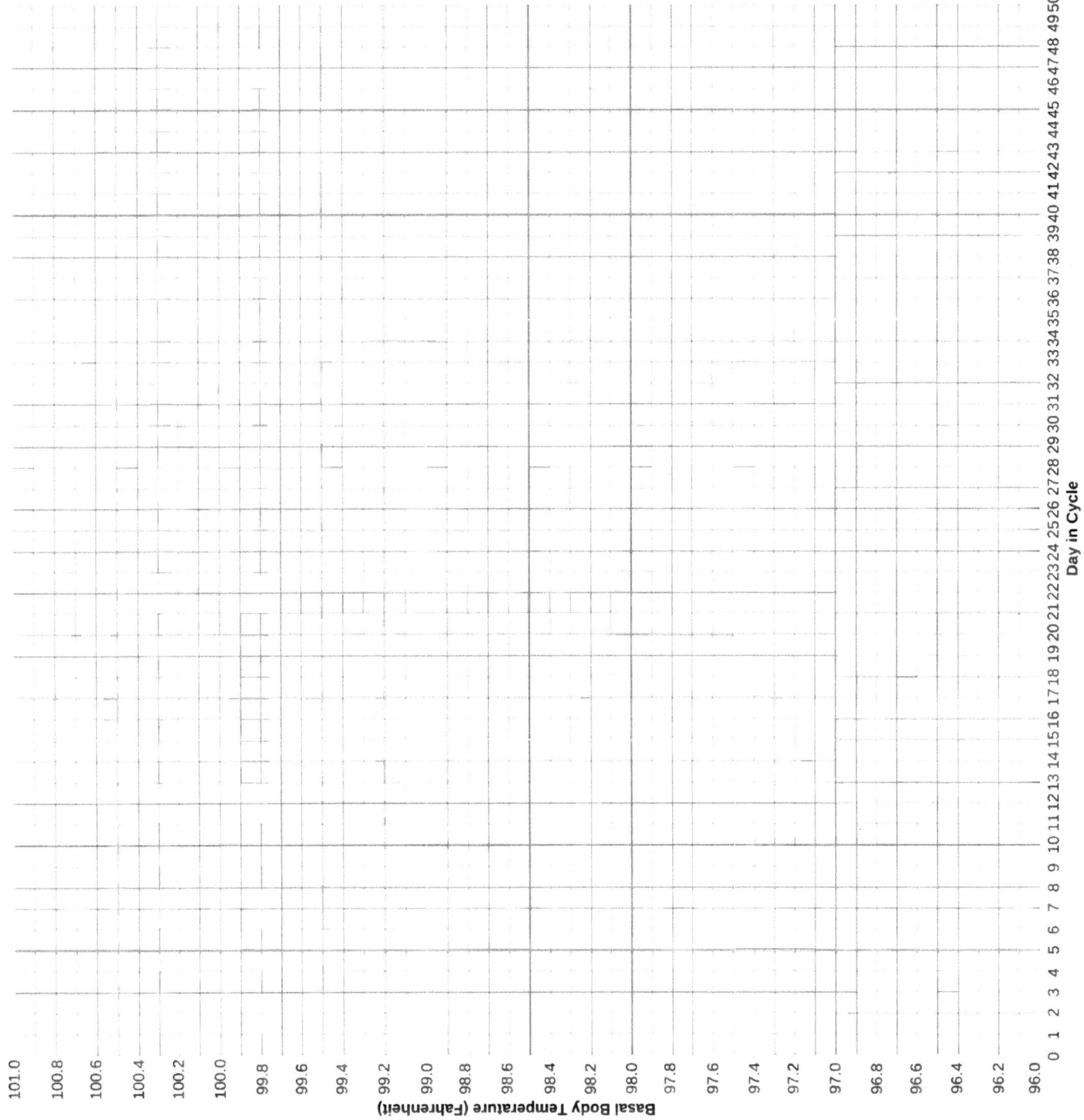

date range _____

cycle # _____

Basal Body Temperature (Fahrenheit)	Day in Cycle
101.0	
100.8	
100.6	
100.4	
100.2	
100.0	
99.8	
99.6	
99.4	
99.2	
99.0	
98.8	
98.6	
98.4	
98.2	
98.0	
97.8	
97.6	
97.4	
97.2	
97.0	
96.8	
96.6	
96.4	
96.2	
96.0	

0 1 2 3 4 5 6 7 8 9 10 11 12 13 14 15 16 17 18 19 20 21 22 23 24 25 26 27 28 29 30 31 32 33 34 35 36 37 38 39 40 41 42 43 44 45 46 47 48 49 50

Day in Cycle

Cycle tracker

first day of period _____

cycle number _____

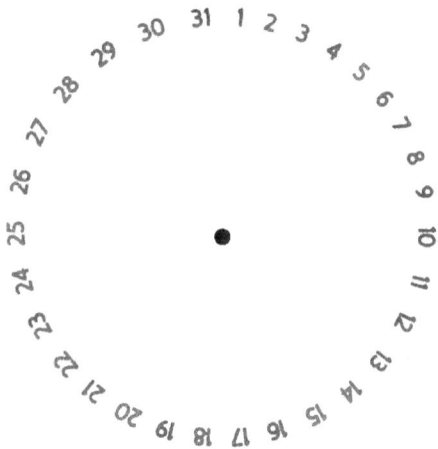

Menstruation Flow

Day 1	Day 2	Day 3
◊◊◊◊◊	◊◊◊◊◊	◊◊◊◊◊

Day 4	Day 5	Day 6
◊◊◊◊◊	◊◊◊◊◊	◊◊◊◊◊

Day 7

◊◊◊◊◊

Mood

Day 1	Day 2	Day 3	Day 4	Day 5	Day 6	Day 7
calm	calm	calm	calm	calm	calm	calm
happy	happy	happy	happy	happy	happy	happy
energetic	energetic	energetic	energetic	energetic	energetic	energetic
irritated	irritated	irritated	irritated	irritated	irritated	irritated
sad	sad	sad	sad	sad	sad	sad
anxious	anxious	anxious	anxious	anxious	anxious	anxious

Symptoms

Day 1	Day 2	Day 3	Day 4	Day 5	Day 6	Day 7
acne	acne	acne	acne	acne	acne	acne
nausea	nausea	nausea	nausea	nausea	nausea	nausea
cramps	cramps	cramps	cramps	cramps	cramps	cramps
headache	headache	headache	headache	headache	headache	headache
fatigue	fatigue	fatigue	fatigue	fatigue	fatigue	fatigue
bloating	bloating	bloating	bloating	bloating	bloating	bloating
back ache	back ache	back ache	back ache	back ache	back ache	back ache
sore boobs	sore boobs	sore boobs	sore boobs	sore boobs	sore boobs	sore boobs

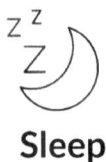

Sleep

_____

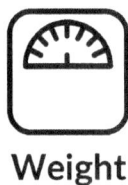

Weight

_____

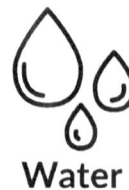

Water

_____

December
1
2
3
4
5
6
7
8
9
10
11
12
13
14
15
16
17
18
19
20
21
22
23
24
25
26
27
28
29
30
31

Notes:

Date _____ # Daily Cycle Log Cycle Day _____

temperature _____ opk result _____ cervical fluid _____
(none, sticky, egg white, watery, unusual)

my mood today is...

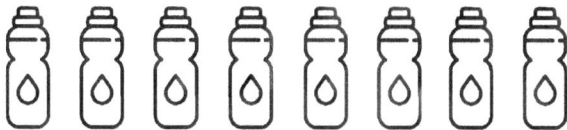

good ☐ fine ☐ so/so ☐ bad ☐ horrible ☐

water intake tracker

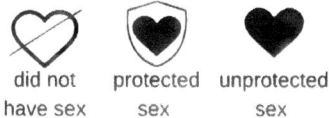

thoughts about how i'm feeling :

_____
_____
_____
_____

exercise

prenatal vitamin 🗂

meals for the day

breakfast _____
lunch _____
dinner _____
snacks _____

Intercourse

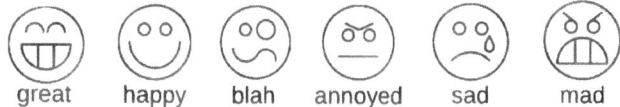

did not have sex   protected sex   unprotected sex

Mood

great   happy   blah   annoyed   sad   mad

Symptoms

tender breasts	headache	backache	fatigue	cravings
cramps	acne	nausea	bloating	insomnia
constipation	diarrhea	joint pain	spotting	congestion

Daily Cycle Log

Date _____   Cycle Day_____

temperature _____   opk result _____   cervical fluid _____
(none, sticky, egg white, watery, unusual)

my mood today is...

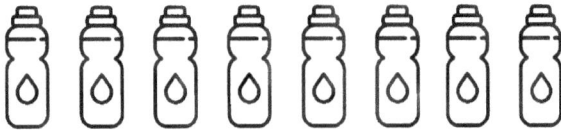

good □   fine □   so/so □   bad □   horrible □

thoughts about how i'm feeling :

_____

_____

_____

_____

exercise

prenatal vitamin

water intake tracker

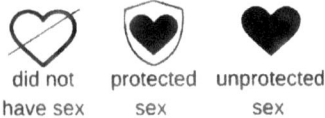

meals for the day

breakfast_____

lunch_____

dinner_____

snacks_____

Intercourse

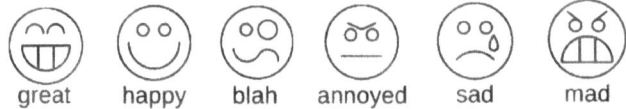

did not have sex   protected sex   unprotected sex

Mood

great   happy   blah   annoyed   sad   mad

Symptoms

tender breasts	headache	backache	fatigue	cravings
cramps	acne	nausea	bloating	insomnia
constipation	diarrhea	joint pain	spotting	congestion

Date _____ # Daily Cycle Log   Cycle Day_____

temperature _____   opk result_____   cervical fluid _____
(none, sticky, egg white, watery, unusual)

my mood today is...

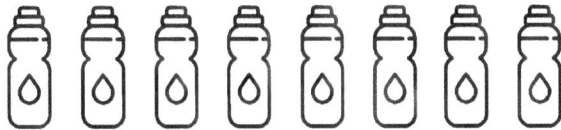

good   *fine*   *so/so*   *bad*   *horrible*
☐   ☐   ☐   ☐   ☐

water intake tracker

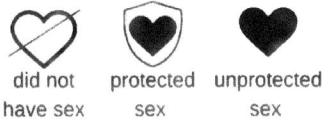

thoughts about how i'm feeling :

_____
_____
_____
_____

exercise

meals for the day

prenatal vitamin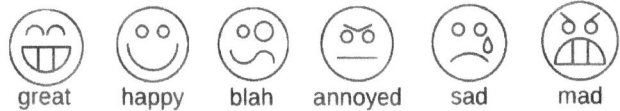

*breakfast*_____

*lunch*_____

*dinner*_____

*snacks*_____

Intercourse

did not   protected   unprotected
have sex   sex   sex

Mood

great   happy   blah   annoyed   sad   mad

Symptoms

tender breasts	headache	backache	fatigue	cravings
cramps	acne	nausea	bloating	insomnia
constipation	diarrhea	joint pain	spotting	congestion

Daily Cycle Log

Date _____

Cycle Day_____

temperature _____   opk result_____   cervical fluid _____
(none, sticky, egg white, watery, unusual)

my mood today is...

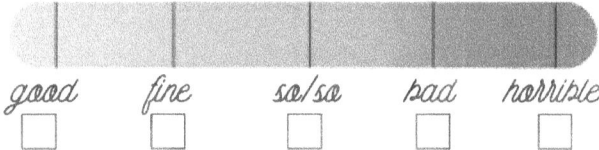

good   fine   so/so   bad   horrible
☐   ☐   ☐   ☐   ☐

thoughts about how i'm feeling :

_____

_____

_____

_____

exercise

water intake tracker

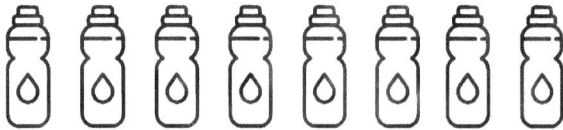

prenatal vitamin ❑❑

meals for the day

breakfast _____

lunch _____

dinner _____

snacks _____

Intercourse

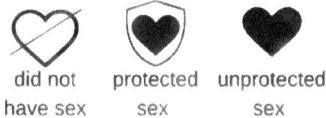

did not have sex   protected sex   unprotected sex

Mood

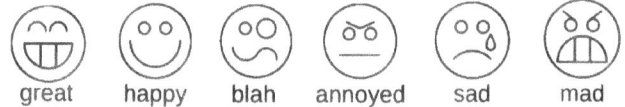

great   happy   blah   annoyed   sad   mad

Symptoms

tender breasts	headache	backache	fatigue	cravings
cramps	acne	nausea	bloating	insomnia
constipation	diarrhea	joint pain	spotting	congestion

Daily Cycle Log

Date _____   Cycle Day_____

temperature _____   opk result _____   cervical fluid _____
(none, sticky, egg white, watery, unusual)

my mood today is...

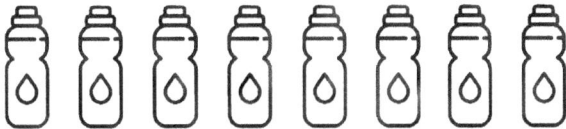

good ☐   fine ☐   so/so ☐   bad ☐   horrible ☐

thoughts about how i'm feeling :

_____

_____

_____

_____

water intake tracker

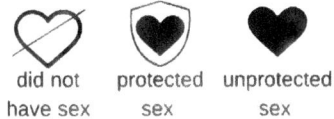

exercise

meals for the day

prenatal vitamin

breakfast _____

lunch _____

dinner _____

snacks _____

Intercourse

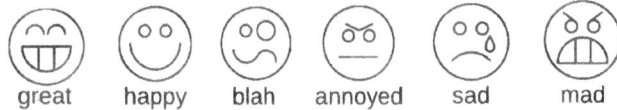

did not have sex   protected sex   unprotected sex

Mood

great   happy   blah   annoyed   sad   mad

Symptoms

tender breasts	headache	backache	fatigue	cravings
cramps	acne	nausea	bloating	insomnia
constipation	diarrhea	joint pain	spotting	congestion

Daily Cycle Log

Date _____   Cycle Day_____

temperature _____   opk result_____   cervical fluid _____
(none, sticky, egg white, watery, unusual)

my mood today is...

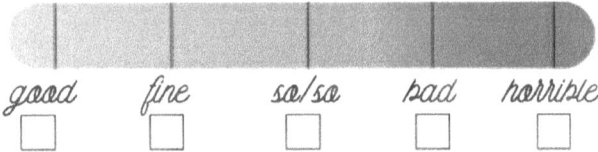

good   *fine*   *so/so*   *bad*   *horrible*
☐   ☐   ☐   ☐   ☐

thoughts about how i'm feeling :

_____

_____

_____

_____

water intake tracker

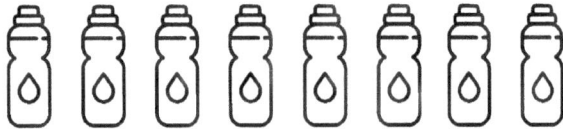

exercise

meals for the day

prenatal vitamin ⧉

*breakfast*_____

*lunch*_____

*dinner*_____

*snacks*_____

Intercourse

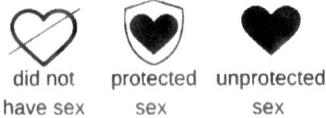

did not   protected   unprotected
have sex   sex   sex

Mood

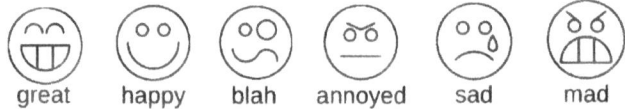

great   happy   blah   annoyed   sad   mad

Symptoms

tender breasts	headache	backache	fatigue	cravings
cramps	acne	nausea	bloating	insomnia
constipation	diarrhea	joint pain	spotting	congestion

Daily Cycle Log

Date _____   Cycle Day _____

temperature _____   opk result _____   cervical fluid _____
(none, sticky, egg white, watery, unusual)

my mood today is...

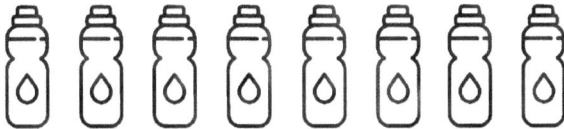

good ☐   fine ☐   so/so ☐   bad ☐   horrible ☐

water intake tracker

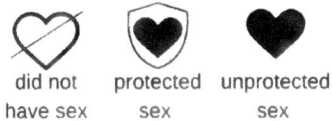

thoughts about how i'm feeling :

_____
_____
_____
_____

exercise
_____
| |
| |
| |
|_____|

prenatal vitamin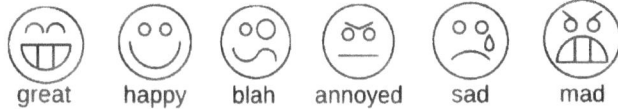

meals for the day

breakfast _____

lunch _____

dinner _____

snacks _____

Intercourse

did not have sex   protected sex   unprotected sex

Mood

great   happy   blah   annoyed   sad   mad

Symptoms

tender breasts	headache	backache	fatigue	cravings
cramps	acne	nausea	bloating	insomnia
constipation	diarrhea	joint pain	spotting	congestion

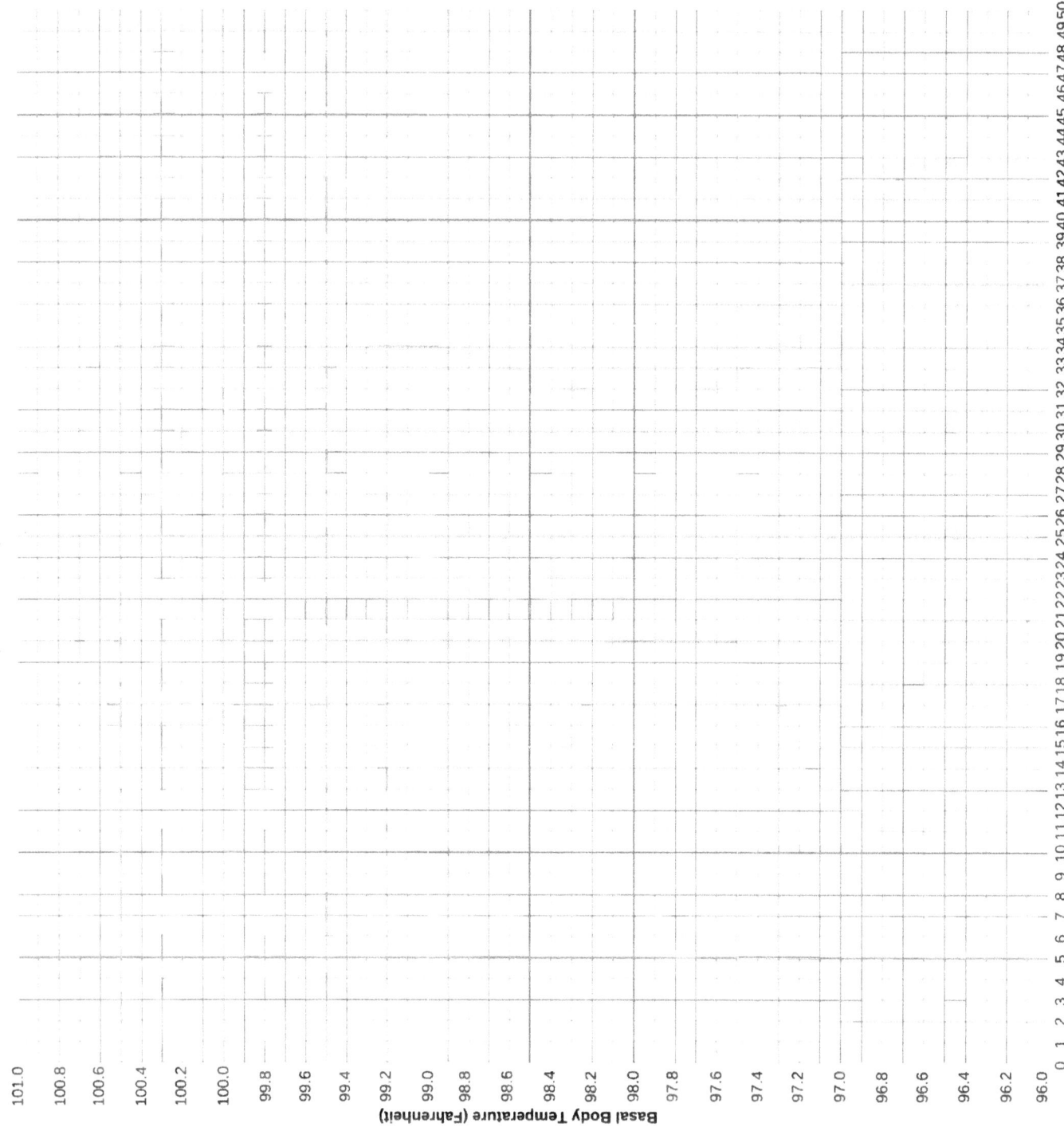

basal body temperature chart

Basal Body Temperature (Fahrenheit)

101.0
100.8
100.6
100.4
100.2
100.0
99.8
99.6
99.4
99.2
99.0
98.8
98.6
98.4
98.2
98.0
97.8
97.6
97.4
97.2
97.0
96.8
96.6
96.4
96.2
96.0

0 1 2 3 4 5 6 7 8 9 10 11 12 13 14 15 16 17 18 19 20 21 22 23 24 25 26 27 28 29 30 31 32 33 34 35 36 37 38 39 40 41 42 43 44 45 46 47 48 49 50

Day in Cycle

Medical Appointment Log

Description: _____

Visit/Call	Date:	Time:

QUESTIONS TO ASK & NOTES

Description: _____

Visit/Call	Date:	Time:

QUESTIONS TO ASK & NOTES

Medical Appointment Log

Description: _____

Visit/Call	Date:	Time:

QUESTIONS TO ASK & NOTES

Description: _____

Visit/Call	Date:	Time:

QUESTIONS TO ASK & NOTES

Medical Appointment Log

Description: _____

Visit/Call	Date:	Time:

QUESTIONS TO ASK & NOTES

Description: _____

Visit/Call	Date:	Time:

QUESTIONS TO ASK & NOTES

Medical Appointment Log

Description: _____

Visit/Call	Date:	Time:

QUESTIONS TO ASK & NOTES

Description: _____

Visit/Call	Date:	Time:

QUESTIONS TO ASK & NOTES

Medical Appointment Log

Description: _____

Visit/Call	Date:	Time:

QUESTIONS TO ASK & NOTES

Description: _____

Visit/Call	Date:	Time:

QUESTIONS TO ASK & NOTES

Medical Appointment Log

Description: _____

Visit/Call	Date:	Time:

QUESTIONS TO ASK & NOTES

Description: _____

Visit/Call	Date:	Time:

QUESTIONS TO ASK & NOTES

Medical Appointment Log

Description: _____

Visit/Call	Date:	Time:

QUESTIONS TO ASK & NOTES

Description: _____

Visit/Call	Date:	Time:

QUESTIONS TO ASK & NOTES

Medical Appointment Log

Description: _____

Visit/Call	Date:	Time:

QUESTIONS TO ASK & NOTES

Description: _____

Visit/Call	Date:	Time:

QUESTIONS TO ASK & NOTES

Medical Appointment Log

Description: _____

Visit/Call	Date:	Time:

QUESTIONS TO ASK & NOTES

Description: _____

Visit/Call	Date:	Time:

QUESTIONS TO ASK & NOTES

Medical Appointment Log

Description: _____

Visit/Call	Date:	Time:

QUESTIONS TO ASK & NOTES

Description: _____

Visit/Call	Date:	Time:

QUESTIONS TO ASK & NOTES

Medication Log

CYCLE:

CD	DATE	TIME	MEDICATION/SUPPLEMENT	DOSE

Medication Log

CYCLE:

CD	DATE	TIME	MEDICATION/SUPPLEMENT	DOSE

Medication Log

CYCLE:

CD	DATE	TIME	MEDICATION/SUPPLEMENT	DOSE

Medication Log

CYCLE:

CD	DATE	TIME	MEDICATION/SUPPLEMENT	DOSE

Medication Log

CYCLE:

CD	DATE	TIME	MEDICATION/SUPPLEMENT	DOSE

WEEKLY PLANNER

WEEK OF:

WEEKLY FOCUS

Sunday

- [ ]
- [ ]
- [ ]
- [ ]
- [ ]

Monday

- [ ]
- [ ]
- [ ]
- [ ]
- [ ]

Tuesday

- [ ]
- [ ]
- [ ]
- [ ]
- [ ]

Wednesday

- [ ]
- [ ]
- [ ]
- [ ]
- [ ]

Thursday

- [ ]
- [ ]
- [ ]
- [ ]
- [ ]

Friday

- [ ]
- [ ]
- [ ]
- [ ]
- [ ]

Saturday

- [ ]
- [ ]
- [ ]
- [ ]
- [ ]

WEEKLY PLANNER

WEEK OF:

WEEKLY FOCUS

Sunday

- [ ]
- [ ]
- [ ]
- [ ]
- [ ]

Monday

- [ ]
- [ ]
- [ ]
- [ ]
- [ ]

Tuesday

- [ ]
- [ ]
- [ ]
- [ ]
- [ ]

Wednesday

- [ ]
- [ ]
- [ ]
- [ ]
- [ ]

Thursday

- [ ]
- [ ]
- [ ]
- [ ]
- [ ]

Friday

- [ ]
- [ ]
- [ ]
- [ ]
- [ ]

Saturday

- [ ]
- [ ]
- [ ]
- [ ]
- [ ]

WEEKLY PLANNER

WEEK OF:

WEEKLY FOCUS

Sunday

- [ ]
- [ ]
- [ ]
- [ ]
- [ ]

Monday

- [ ]
- [ ]
- [ ]
- [ ]
- [ ]

Tuesday

- [ ]
- [ ]
- [ ]
- [ ]
- [ ]

Wednesday

- [ ]
- [ ]
- [ ]
- [ ]
- [ ]

Thursday

- [ ]
- [ ]
- [ ]
- [ ]
- [ ]

Friday

- [ ]
- [ ]
- [ ]
- [ ]
- [ ]

Saturday

- [ ]
- [ ]
- [ ]
- [ ]
- [ ]

WEEKLY PLANNER

WEEK OF:

WEEKLY FOCUS

Sunday

- [ ]
- [ ]
- [ ]
- [ ]
- [ ]

Monday

- [ ]
- [ ]
- [ ]
- [ ]
- [ ]

Tuesday

- [ ]
- [ ]
- [ ]
- [ ]
- [ ]

Wednesday

- [ ]
- [ ]
- [ ]
- [ ]
- [ ]

Thursday

- [ ]
- [ ]
- [ ]
- [ ]
- [ ]

Friday

- [ ]
- [ ]
- [ ]
- [ ]
- [ ]

Saturday

- [ ]
- [ ]
- [ ]
- [ ]
- [ ]

WEEKLY PLANNER

WEEK OF:

WEEKLY FOCUS

Sunday

- [ ]
- [ ]
- [ ]
- [ ]
- [ ]

Monday

- [ ]
- [ ]
- [ ]
- [ ]
- [ ]

Tuesday

- [ ]
- [ ]
- [ ]
- [ ]
- [ ]

Wednesday

- [ ]
- [ ]
- [ ]
- [ ]
- [ ]

Thursday

- [ ]
- [ ]
- [ ]
- [ ]
- [ ]

Friday

- [ ]
- [ ]
- [ ]
- [ ]
- [ ]

Saturday

- [ ]
- [ ]
- [ ]
- [ ]
- [ ]

WEEKLY PLANNER

WEEK OF:

WEEKLY FOCUS

Sunday

Monday

Tuesday

Wednesday

Thursday

Friday

Saturday

WEEKLY PLANNER

WEEK OF:

WEEKLY FOCUS

Sunday

- [ ]
- [ ]
- [ ]
- [ ]
- [ ]

Monday

- [ ]
- [ ]
- [ ]
- [ ]
- [ ]

Tuesday

- [ ]
- [ ]
- [ ]
- [ ]
- [ ]

Wednesday

- [ ]
- [ ]
- [ ]
- [ ]
- [ ]

Thursday

- [ ]
- [ ]
- [ ]
- [ ]
- [ ]

Friday

- [ ]
- [ ]
- [ ]
- [ ]
- [ ]

Saturday

- [ ]
- [ ]
- [ ]
- [ ]
- [ ]

WEEKLY PLANNER

WEEK OF:

WEEKLY FOCUS

Sunday

- [ ]
- [ ]
- [ ]
- [ ]
- [ ]

Monday

- [ ]
- [ ]
- [ ]
- [ ]
- [ ]

Tuesday

- [ ]
- [ ]
- [ ]
- [ ]
- [ ]

Wednesday

- [ ]
- [ ]
- [ ]
- [ ]
- [ ]

Thursday

- [ ]
- [ ]
- [ ]
- [ ]
- [ ]

Friday

- [ ]
- [ ]
- [ ]
- [ ]
- [ ]

Saturday

- [ ]
- [ ]
- [ ]
- [ ]
- [ ]

WEEKLY PLANNER

WEEK OF:

WEEKLY FOCUS

Sunday

- [ ]
- [ ]
- [ ]
- [ ]
- [ ]

Monday

- [ ]
- [ ]
- [ ]
- [ ]
- [ ]

Tuesday

- [ ]
- [ ]
- [ ]
- [ ]
- [ ]

Wednesday

- [ ]
- [ ]
- [ ]
- [ ]
- [ ]

Thursday

- [ ]
- [ ]
- [ ]
- [ ]

Friday

- [ ]
- [ ]
- [ ]
- [ ]
- [ ]

Saturday

- [ ]
- [ ]
- [ ]
- [ ]
- [ ]

WEEKLY PLANNER

WEEK OF:

WEEKLY FOCUS

Sunday

- [ ]
- [ ]
- [ ]
- [ ]
- [ ]

Monday

- [ ]
- [ ]
- [ ]
- [ ]
- [ ]

Tuesday

- [ ]
- [ ]
- [ ]
- [ ]
- [ ]

Wednesday

- [ ]
- [ ]
- [ ]
- [ ]
- [ ]

Thursday

- [ ]
- [ ]
- [ ]
- [ ]
- [ ]

Friday

- [ ]
- [ ]
- [ ]
- [ ]
- [ ]

Saturday

- [ ]
- [ ]
- [ ]
- [ ]
- [ ]

WEEKLY PLANNER

WEEK OF:

WEEKLY FOCUS

Sunday
- [ ]
- [ ]
- [ ]
- [ ]
- [ ]

Monday
- [ ]
- [ ]
- [ ]
- [ ]
- [ ]

Tuesday
- [ ]
- [ ]
- [ ]
- [ ]
- [ ]

Wednesday
- [ ]
- [ ]
- [ ]
- [ ]
- [ ]

Thursday
- [ ]
- [ ]
- [ ]
- [ ]
- [ ]

Friday
- [ ]
- [ ]
- [ ]
- [ ]
- [ ]

Saturday
- [ ]
- [ ]
- [ ]
- [ ]
- [ ]

WEEKLY PLANNER

WEEK OF:

WEEKLY FOCUS

Sunday

-
-
-
-
-

Monday

-
-
-
-
-

Tuesday

-
-
-
-
-

Wednesday

-
-
-
-
-

Thursday

-
-
-
-
-

Friday

-
-
-
-
-

Saturday

-
-
-
-
-

NOTES:

Date:

NOTES:

Date:

NOTES:

Date:

NOTES:

Date:

NOTES:

Date:

NOTES:

Date:

NOTES:

Date:

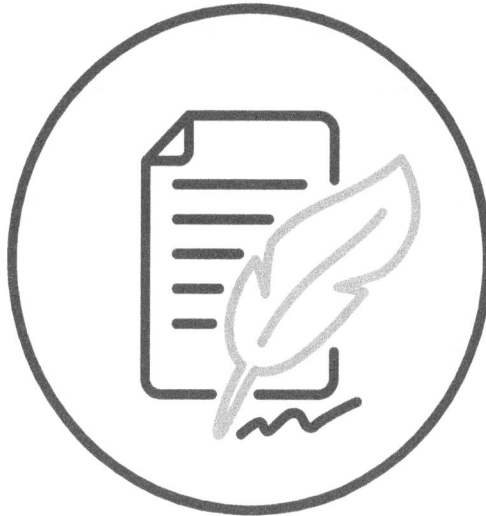

CREATEPUBLICATION

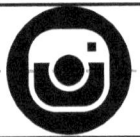

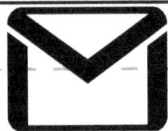

Thank you!

As a small family company, your feedback is very important to us.

Please let us know how you like our book at:

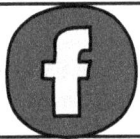

f /createpublication

◎ /createpublication

✉ createpublication@gmail.com

www.ingramcontent.com/pod-product-compliance
Lightning Source LLC
Chambersburg PA
CBHW052113020426

42335CB00021B/2739